Andrew Lieberman

RENAL DIET FISH, SEAFOOD AND MEAT RECIPES

UNDERSTANDING KIDNEY DISEASE AND AVOID DIALYSIS

52 Fish, Seafood and Meat Recipes

TABLE OF CONTENTS

—

4

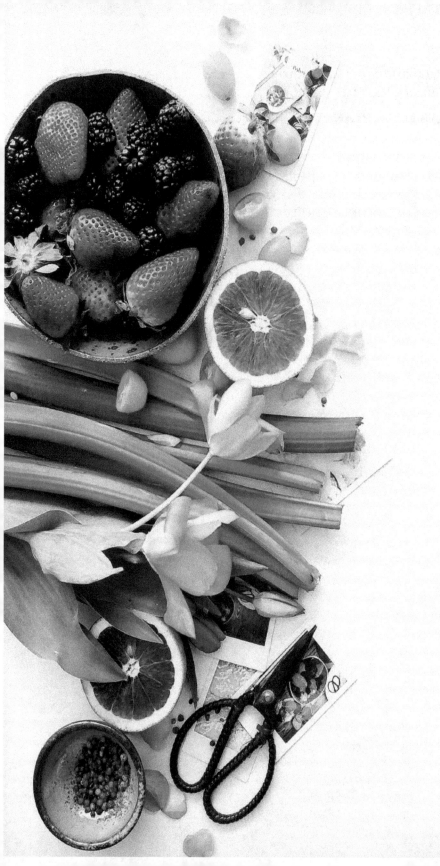

O ne way to prevent kidney disease is with a proper diet. It's also important to know that those at risk of this disease or have already been diagnosed with this condition can help alleviate symptoms and slow down the disease's progression with a diet called the renal diet. As you know, the wastes in the blood come from the foods and drinks that you consume. Scraps that remain in the blood can negatively affect your overall health. Following a renal diet can help bolster the kidney's functioning, reduce damage to the kidneys, and prevent kidney failure.

A renal diet is a type of diet that involves consuming foods and drinks that are low in potassium, sodium, and phosphorus.

It also focuses on the consumption of high-quality protein and limiting too much intake of fluids and calcium. Since each person's body is different, it's essential to develop a specific diet formulated by a dietician to make sure that the diet is tailored to the patient's needs. Some of the substances you have to check and monitor for proper renal diet include The Benefits of Renal Diet. A renal diet minimizes the intake of sodium, potassium, and phosphorus. Excessive sodium is harmful to people who have been diagnosed with kidney disease, as this causes fluid buildup, making it hard for the kidneys to eliminate sodium and fluid. Improper functioning of the kidneys can also mean difficulty in removing excess potassium. Kidneys that are not working find it difficult to remove excess phosphorus correctly.

There are many benefits to adapting to the renal diet, whether you have kidney disease or related conditions. It's an excellent way to eat and live, especially if you may be susceptible to kidney infections and other issues that impact this vital organ's function. It includes making changes early and paying close attention to your symptoms and any changes you notice. These may indicate the progression itself or a positive change in your kidneys' function in the disease. Keeping an eye on the slightest changes can make a significant difference in improving your health and taking charge of your well-being.

The renal diet focuses primarily on supporting kidney health, but in doing so, you'll improve many other aspects of your health, as well. It can also be customized to kidney disease levels, from early stages and minor infections to more significant renal impairment and dialysis. Preventing the later stages is the primary goal, though reaching this stage can still be treated carefully considering your dietary choices. In addition to medical treatment, the diet provides a way for you to control your health and progression. It can mean the difference between a complete renal failure or a manageable chronic condition, where you can lead a regular, enjoyable life despite having kidney issues.

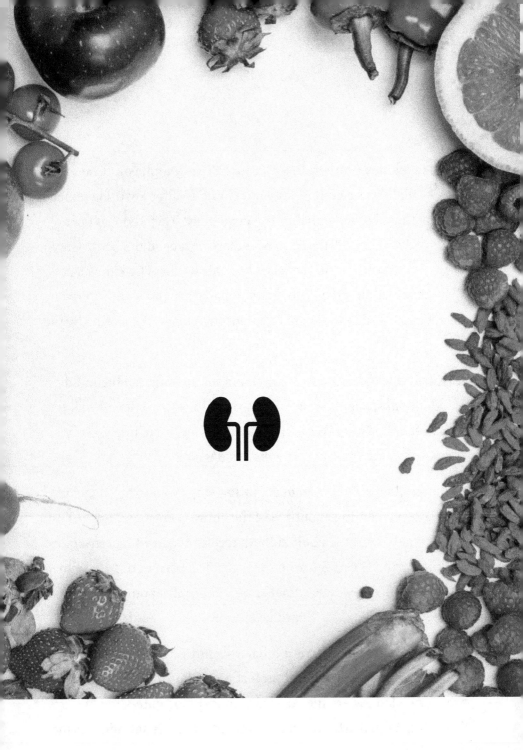

Chapter 1: Understanding Kidney Disease

T he kidneys' importance cannot be over-emphasized, so much that the Ancient Egyptians refused to alter anything about them before embalming a dead body. They did, having no idea of the real functions of these organs in the body. Only the kidneys and the heart had this honor. The kidneys got ascribed the role of advisory to the heart and were revered by the ancients. The kidneys are recipients of a long-time doting by the human race.

Structurally, the two bean-shaped organs are situated behind the abdominal space. They are about 11 centimeters in length. Like every other body part occurring in pairs, they are of unequal sizes, latching onto both sides' spine.

In males, the kidneys weigh about 125 – 175 g and 115 – 155 g in females, representing about 1 % of the entire body mass. Regardless of their small sizes, the adult kidneys receive the most massive blood volume anybody can get from the heart. It is about 20-25 % of the total output. However, a fetal kidney gets only about 2 % of the cardiac output.

Surrounding each organ is a renal capsule and two layers of fatty tissues, serving as a means of protection to the kidneys. Located on top of each kidney are the adrenal glands. Blood enters the kidneys through the renal arteries and is emptied via the renal veins. Urine, the kidneys' primary waste, gets drained into the bladder through the ureter, a tube-like structure.

The kidney is structurally divided into two segments, namely the cortex and the medulla. Dispersed between the two parts are approximately a million nephrons. The nephrons are responsible for the urine production and general excretion activity of the kidney via the glomerulus, proximal, and distal tubule.

Glomerular filtration: The process is thus named because it takes place in the glomerulus part of the nephron before passing into the Bowman's capsule. The kidneys daily produce about 180 liters' filtrates using a combination of charge and size selection. Therefore, molecules of excessive charges or big sizes will not pass through the filter. Proteins of large dimensions and red blood cells, therefore, do not undergo filtration.

The filtration rate of human kidneys is not constant over time. The kidneys can adapt to different stages of life. At birth, the glomerular filtration rate is only approximately 10 % of the adult range, but this normalizes by 1. A reabsorption process takes place further down in the tubules, releasing an end product of 1.5 liters' urine, containing a mere one percent of the total filtrate volume. The presence of albumin and red blood cells in excreted urine suggests a damaged glomerulus.

Another name for glomerular filtration is hydrostatic filtration. Three factors affecting the glomerular filtration rate include the hydrostatic pressure, the pore sizes, and the pressure exerted by the colloids. The glomerular filtration rate is essential in the determination of the optimal working of the kidney. The differences in GFR for individuals remain relatively constant as the body finds a means to balance the glomeruli and the pores' sizes.

Even at that, big-sized glomeruli are probable signs of high levels of risk for chronic kidney disease development. Individuals with gross obesity, low birth weight, heart-related diseases, and hypertension may fall into this category. The number of functional nephrons also decreases with age as the glomeruli become hardened.

Secretion: As the name implies, it involves moving out of wastes from the blood into the urine for proper excretion. While reabsorption occurs by a system of passive transport, secretion takes place by active transport. Substances moved out include xenobiotics and some ions. The proximal tubule is the location for secretion.

The proximal tubule is the first point for reabsorption of nutrients back into the body. About 55 percent of fluid is reabsorbed into the body in this area. Nutrients and minerals migrate from a high concentration in the tubules to the lower concentrated capillaries outside. No glucose escapes this stage at an optimal plasma concentration.

However, an increased plasma level is an indicator of diabetes as sugar can pass through with urine from the kidney, a condition known as glycosuria. The total reabsorption of amino acids also occurs in the proximal tubules through dedicated transporters. Other minerals reabsorbed in the proximal tubules are sodium, chloride, bicarbonate, water, and phosphate. Other reabsorption points are the loop of Henle, the distal tubules, and then the collecting tubules.

By the time the filtrate reaches the last checkpoint of reabsorption, almost 99 % of filtrate would have been reabsorbed. A urea-concentrated waste is the end product of this phase. The collecting tubules serve as the link between the nephrons and the immediate surrounding environment, the ureter.

Wastes move out of the nephrons through the collecting tubules into the renal pelvis. This process is called excretion. One primary factor affecting reabsorption is the pH of urine. Alkaline urine leads to a greater rate of excretion and vice versa.

The kidney is also responsible for the regulation of blood pressure. A loss of kidney function is closely and directly related to high blood pressure. The renal glands' operation on blood pressure is cumulative, showing results only in the long term. However, its effects are the most prominent and require careful observation.

The human blood pressure is regulated via several systems, one of which is the renin-angiotensin-aldosterone system (RAAS), mediated by several different hormones. The kidney produces renin using juxtaglomerular cells. It is dependent on several signals, such as fluctuations in blood pressure, sodium levels, and the nervous system.

The secreted renin is then converted into angiotensin I, which goes through a further transformation to form angiotensin II that increases arterial pressure. The summary of the RAAS's long process is the regulation of the sodium present in the blood to maintain arteriole pressure. There is a relationship between the hormone renin, angiotensin, aldosterone, and blood pressure. Some of the noticeable signs during high blood pressure are the following:

Ø Vasoconstriction of the body's arterioles

Ø Increased rate of sodium reabsorption into the blood

Ø Production and secretion of antidiuretic hormone and aldosterone, all acting to increase the blood pressure of the body

The renal organ's urine synthesis shows that the kidneys are also responsible for maintaining the ratio of water to some other electrolytes (salts) in the body through the secretion of the antidiuretic hormones. There is a relationship between the hormone and salt reabsorption. This function remains crucial too in the control of blood pressure.

The renal glands also help to maintain the pH of the blood along with the lungs. Here, our diet has some roles to play. The consumption of protein-rich foods leads to the production of acidic urine and vice-versa. The kidneys and lungs strive to keep the blood's pH around neutral such that it is neither acidic nor basic.

Apart from the kidney's regulatory roles, it is also involved in the production of some hormones such as rennin, erythropoietin, antidiuretic hormone, and calcitriol.

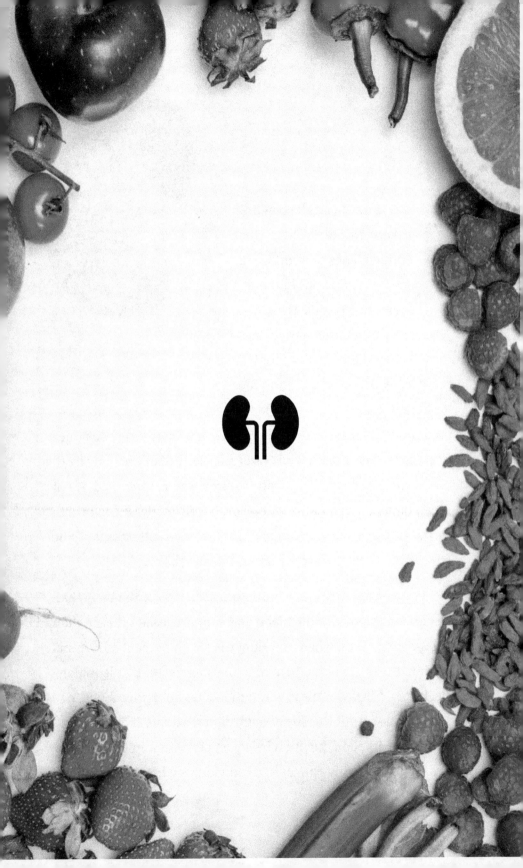

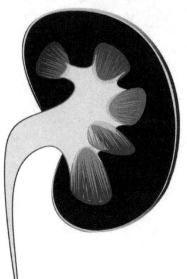

How is our health depending on our kidneys? That's what often comes to mind when we overlook our kidneys' function or take them for granted. Imagine waste produced and released into your blood is removed continuously around the clock—and not only that but the kidneys are also responsible for maintaining the fluids and water levels in the body. You consume a lot of excess water, then the excess is released out of the body by the kidneys, and in case of dehydration, more water is retained. All of this can happen if the kidneys are working correctly. It can lead to toxic buildup in the body, damaging kidneys and other organs and disturbing the natural metabolism.

Most people are born with a kidney on each side of the body that simultaneously purifies the blood and supports each other in their renal function. Even when one kidney loses 40 percent of its renal function, the other kidney can hide this damage until adequately checked and tested. This is why patients do not know about the renal disease until there is enough damage done. If any of the kidneys lose its renal function below 25 percent, it must raise the alarms, which is highly dangerous. Individuals whose renal function decreases to only 15 percent would require an external treatment or dialysis.

Chronic kidney disease is a slow-moving disease and does not cause the patient many complaints in the initial stages. The group of chronic kidney disease diseases includes several kidney diseases, in which case the renal function decreases for several years or decades. With the help of timely diagnosis and treatment can slow down and even stop kidney disease progression.

In international studies of renal function in many people, it was found that almost every tenth kidney was found to have impaired kidney function to one degree or another.

Chronic kidney disease can be present at any age. The most significant risk of getting sick is in people who have one or more of the following risk factors:

- Diabetes
- High blood pressure
- Family members have previously had kidney disease.
- Age over 50
- Long-term consumption of drugs that can damage the kidneys
- Overweight or obesity

What are the Symptoms of Chronic Kidney Disease?

If chronic kidney disease progresses, then the blood levels of end products of metabolism increase, which is the cause of feeling unwell. Various health problems may occur, such as high blood pressure, anemia (anemia), bone disease, premature cardiovascular calcification, discoloration, composition, and urine volume.

As the disease progresses, the main symptoms can be:

- Weakness, the feeling of weakness
- Dyspnea
- Trouble sleeping
- Lack of appetite
- Dry skin, itchy skin
- Muscle cramps, especially at night
- Swelling in the legs
- Swelling eyes, especially in the morning.

Diagnose with Chronic Kidney Disease

There are two simple tests that your family doctor can prescribe to diagnose kidney disease.

- Blood test: glomerular filtration rate (GFR) and serum creatinine level. Creatinine is one of those end products of protein metabolism. The blood level depends on age, gender, muscle mass, nutrition, physical activity, on which foods before taking the sample (for example, a lot of meat was eaten), and some drugs. Creatinine is excreted from the body through the kidneys, and if the work of the kidneys slows down, creatinine blood plasma increases. Determining the creatinine level alone is insufficient for diagnosing chronic kidney disease since its value begins to exceed the upper limit of the norm only when GFR decreased by half. GFR is calculated using four parameters that consider the patient's creatinine reading, age, gender, and race. GFR shows at what level is the ability of the kidneys to filter. In chronic kidney disease, the GFR indicator indicates the stage of the severity of kidney disease.

- Urine analysis: the content of albumin in the urine is determined; also, the values of albumin and creatinine in the urine are determined by each other. Albumin is a protein in the urine that usually enters the urine in minimal quantities. Even a small increase in the level of albumin in the urine in some people may be an early sign of incipient kidney disease, especially in those with diabetes and high blood pressure. In normal kidney function, albumin in the urine should be no more than 3 mg/moll (or 30 mg g). If albumin excretion increases even more, then it already speaks of kidney disease. If albumin excretion exceeds 300 mg g, other proteins are excreted into the urine, and this condition is called proteinuria.

If the kidney is healthy, then albumin does not enter the urine.

In the case of an injured kidney, albumin begins to enter the urine.

If the doctor suspects that there is a kidney disease after receiving the urine analysis results, then an additional urine analysis is performed for albumin. If it is detected again within three months, then this indicates chronic kidney disease.

ADDITIONAL EXAMINATIONS

In kidney ultrasound examination: in the diagnosis of chronic kidney disease, it is an examination of the primary choice. Ultrasound examination allows assessing the kidneys' shape, size, location and determines possible changes in the kidney tissue and other abnormalities that may interfere with the kidneys' normal functioning. Ultrasound examination of the kidneys does not require special training and has no risks for the patient.

If necessary, and if a urological disease is suspected, an ultrasound examination of the urinary tract can be prescribed (as well as a residual urine analysis). An ultrasound examination of the prostate gland can be prescribed for men and referred to a urologist for a consultation. If necessary, and if a disease is suspected, a woman is referred for consultation to a gynecologist.

You need to know about the examination with a contrast agent. If you have chronic kidney disease, diagnostic tests such as magnetic resonance imaging, computed tomography, and angiography are used to diagnose and treat various diseases and injuries. In many cases, intravenous and intra-arterial contrast agents (containing iodine or gadolinium) are used, making it possible to see the organs or blood vessels under study.

What is particularly important to do before the survey pole to gain in contrast substance?

If you are scheduled for an examination with a contrast agent, you need to determine your GFR.

Together with your doctor, you can discuss and evaluate the benefits or harm to your health. If the survey is still necessary, follow the following preparation rules:

The day before the survey and the day after the survey, drink plenty of fluids (water, tea, etc.). If you are on treatment in a hospital, you will be injected with the necessary fluid through a vein by infusion. When staying in hospital treatment after examination with a contrast agent (within 48-96 hours), it is usually prescribed to determine creatinine's level in the blood to assess renal function. In the outpatient examination with a contrast agent, your family doctor will be able to evaluate your kidney function.

Discuss with your doctor the questions about which medications should not be taken before examining a contrast agent. Some drugs (antibiotics, drugs against high blood pressure, etc.) and contrasting substances begin to act as a poison. The day before and the day after the examination, in no case should you take metformin - a cure for diabetes.

Between the two examinations with a contrast agent, at the first opportunity, sufficient time should be left for the contrast agent that was used during the first examination to leave the body. It is essential to exclude repeated studies with a large amount of contrast material.

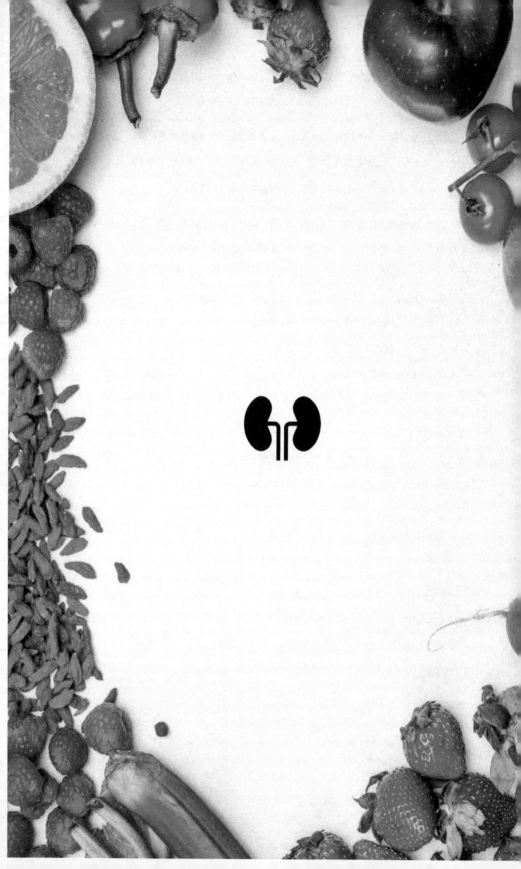

A renal diet minimizes the intake of sodium, potassium, and phosphorus.

Improper functioning of the kidneys can also mean difficulty in removing excess potassium.

When there is too much potassium in the body, this can lead to hyperkalemia, which can also cause problems with the heart and blood vessels.

Kidneys that are not working find it difficult to remove excess phosphorus efficiently.

High levels of phosphorus excrete calcium from the bones causing them to weaken. It also causes the elevation of calcium deposits in the eyes, heart, lungs, and blood vessels.

WHAT TO EAT AND AVOID IN RENAL DIET

A renal diet focuses on natural and nutritious foods, but at the same time, are low in sodium, potassium, and phosphorus.

FOODS TO EAT:

- Cauliflower - 1 cup contains 19 mg sodium, 176 potassium, 40 mg phosphorus
- Blueberries - 1 cup contains 1.5 mg sodium, 114 potassium, 18 mg phosphorus
- Sea Bass - 3 ounces contain 74 mg sodium, 279 potassium, 211 mg phosphorus
- Grapes - 1/2 cup contains 1.5 mg sodium, 144 potassium, 15 mg phosphorus
- Egg Whites - 2 egg whites contain 110 mg sodium, 108 potassium, 10 mg phosphorus
- Garlic - 3 cloves contain 1.5 mg sodium, 36 potassium, 14 mg phosphorus
- Buckwheat - ½ cup contains 3.5 mg sodium, 74 potassium, 59 mg phosphorus
- Olive Oil - 1 ounce 0.6 mg sodium, 0.3 potassium, 0 mg phosphorus
- Bulgur - ½ cup contains 4.5 mg sodium, 62 potassium, 36 mg phosphorus
- Cabbage - 1 cup contains 13 mg sodium, 119 potassium, 18 mg phosphorus
- Skinless chicken - 3 ounces contain 63 mg sodium, 216 potassium, 192 mg phosphorus
- Bell peppers - 1 piece contains 3 mg sodium, 156 potassium, 19 mg phosphorus.
- Onion - 1 piece contains 3 mg sodium, 102 potassium, 20 mg phosphorus

- Arugula - 1 cup contains 6 mg sodium, 74 potassium, 10 mg phosphorus
- Macadamia nuts - 1 ounce contains 1.4 mg sodium, 103 potassium, 53 mg phosphorus
- Radish - ½ cup contains 23 mg sodium, 135 potassium, 12 mg phosphorus
- Turnips - ½ cup contains 12.5 mg sodium, 138 potassium, 20 mg phosphorus
- Pineapple - 1 cup contains 2 mg sodium, 180 potassium, 13 mg phosphorus
- Cranberries – 1 cup contains 2 mg sodium, 85 potassium, 13 mg phosphorus
- Mushrooms – 1 cup contains 6 mg sodium, 170 potassium, 42 mg phosphorus

FOODS TO AVOID

These foods are known to have high levels of potassium, sodium, or phosphorus:

- Soda – Soda is believed to contain up to 100 mg of additive phosphorus per 200 ml.
- Avocados - 1 cup contains up to 727 mg of potassium.
- Canned foods – Canned foods contain high amounts of sodium, so ensure that you avoid using these or opt for low-sodium versions.
- Whole wheat bread – 1 ounce of bread contains 57 mg phosphorus and 69 mg potassium, higher than white bread.

- Brown rice – 1 cup of brown rice contains 154 mg potassium, while 1 cup of white rice only has 54 mg potassium.
- Bananas – 1 banana contains 422 mg of potassium.
- Dairy – Dairy products are high in potassium, phosphorus, and calcium. You can still consume dairy products, but you have to limit it. Use dairy milk alternatives like almond milk and coconut milk.
- Processed Meats – Processed meats are not advisable for people with kidney problems because of their high content of additives and preservatives.
- Pickled and cured foods – These are made using large amounts of salt.
- Apricots – 1 cup contains 427 mg potassium.
- Potatoes and sweet potatoes – 1 potato contain 610 mg potassium. You can double boil potatoes and sweet potatoes to reduce potassium by 50 percent.
- Tomatoes – 1 cup tomato sauce contains up to 900 mg potassium.
- Instant meals – Instant meals are known for too high amounts of sodium.
- Spinach – Spinach contains up to 290 mg potassium per cup. Cooking helps reduce the amount of potassium.
- Raisins, prunes, and dates – Dried fruits have concentrated nutrients, including potassium. 1 cup of prunes contains up to 1,274 mg potassium.
- Chips – Chips are known to have high amounts of sodium.

BENEFITS OF THE RENAL DIET

Since the Renal Diet is generally a Low Sodium, Low Phosphorus program, there are certain health benefits that you will enjoy from this diet. (Apart from improving your kidney health). Some of the vital ones are below:

- It helps to lower blood pressure.
- It helps to lower your LDL cholesterol.
- It helps to lower your risk of having a heart attack.
- It helps to prevent heart failure.
- It decreases the possibility of having a stroke.
- It helps to protect your vision.
- It helps to improve your memory.
- It helps to lower the possibility of dementia.
- It helps to build stronger bones.

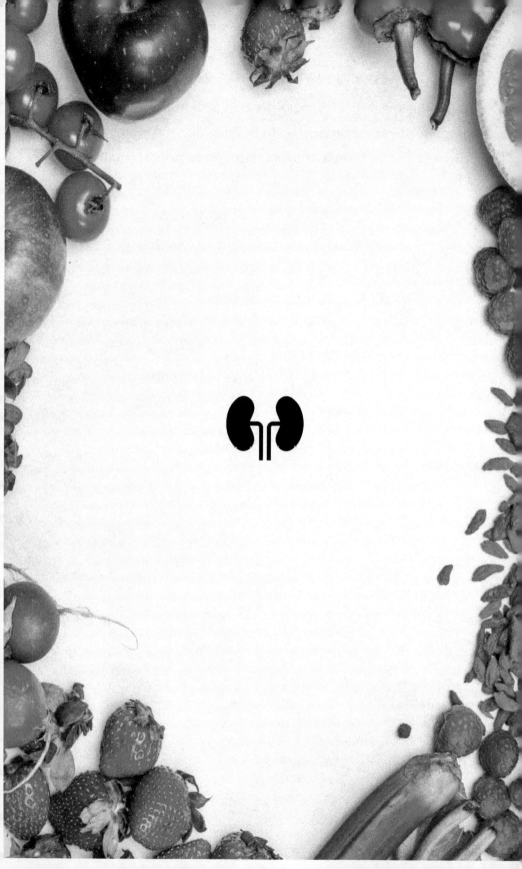

N obody likes restrictions. And if you're used to cooking a certain way, suddenly being faced with a new list of rules can intimidate even the most experienced chef. You'll quickly realize that it is possible to enjoy meals—perhaps more than ever before—regardless of the recommended limitations imposed by renal complications. A basic strategy for sticking with a kidney-healthy diet is to be aware of the nutrient content in your meals and the types of nutrients you may need to limit. For example, you'll be looking to choose foods with less sodium and the right kinds of protein.

You'll see that while these rules are beneficial for slowing the progression of kidney damage, they are healthy for the general population, as well. So, by all means, include your family in your health-supportive menu planning. Lowering sodium intake, for example, will decrease anyone's risk for high blood pressure, while choosing better protein options will reduce saturated fat intake for all diners and, in turn, limit the chances of developing atherosclerosis and heart disease.

To keep the body functioning correctly, we all require essential macronutrients such as fat, carbohydrates, protein, and micronutrients such as sodium and potassium. Being on the renal diet does not change this fundamental fact. However, it does alter the amounts of certain nutrients that the body can tolerate and process. For example, did you know that one teaspoon of table salt equals 2,300 milligrams of sodium? It is already the maximum amount a person should consume in one day!

THE LOW-SODIUM RENAL DIET MEAL PLAN

Many of the essential dietary principles on the renal diet are related to the fluid. The kidneys' inability to excrete fluid also means that water-soluble nutrients can build up in the body and cause harmful effects. Certain nutrients, such as sodium, can cause the body to retain fluid, increase blood pressure, and place added stress on the heart.

There are several ways to limit sodium intake while maintaining a flavorful diet. Less than 2,300 milligrams of sodium (1 teaspoon) should be consumed per day. It may sound not very easy if you're accustomed to keeping a saltshaker on your table, but there are plenty of substitutions that can be made for old-fashioned table salt. For example, substituting dried herbs and seasoning, such as basil and oregano, can maximize flavor without sodium (see Dump the Salt: Explore Your Options, here). Keep in mind that there may be sodium hiding in certain store-bought products, so make sure to check the nutrition labels. Also, watch out for unwanted sodium in canned or frozen foods. A straightforward trick is to rinse your canned vegetables or beans before eating them, eliminating a significant amount of sodium from the food item. If you buy frozen dinners, look for the low-sodium varieties. But without a doubt, purchase fresh, whole foods as often as possible is the best way to control what you are putting in your body.

DUMP THE SALT: EXPLORE YOUR OPTIONS

The science is precise: sodium is of no help to kidneys that are working hard already. But a little experimenting will have you kicking the salt habit as you discover flavorful alternatives that can become your new go-to seasonings. Try some of these tasty, healthier flavor boosters on your meats, grains, and veggies:

- Beer or wine (use sparingly)
- Cardamom
- Cayenne pepper
- Cilantro
- Cinnamon
- Dill
- Garlic and olive oil (just a small bit of oil will fill your dish with flavor!)
- Lemon
- Rosemary
- Scallions, leeks, onions
- Vinegar (there are countless varieties available)

Don't let the list stop here! The supermarket is packed with excellent fresh and dried herbs and spices. One caution: Beware of packaged salt substitutes and spice blends that may contain added salt. The best route is always to create your blend from the ingredients you've chosen.

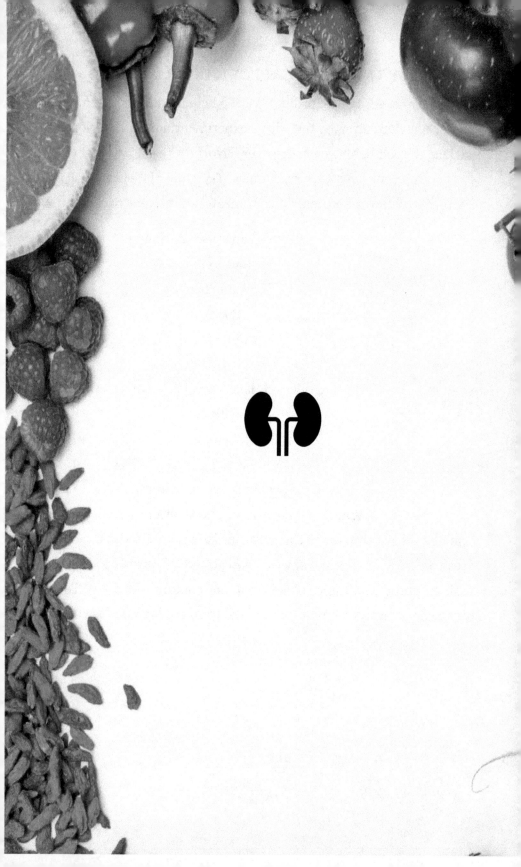

CHAPTER 5: A KIDNEY-FRIENDLY LIFESTYLE

Y ou would vow to stick to a fitness routine at least once every year. However, if you have had some difficulties with the follow-through, you are definitely in good company. Yet there are so many motives for making the commitment and continuing with it again.

Everybody's got a different excuse to lose momentum. The bottom line is to start a workout routine if staying healthy is essential to you. And it takes less time than to navigate down the Facebook page; one may fit in a day's work out.

Possibly, when you watch TV, you should do it if you follow organizations such as the ACE (American Council on Exercise) and CDC (Centers for Disease Control & Prevention).

A full of 150 minutes of exercise per week is what you need to boost your cardiac well-being and decrease your chance of all forms of other diseases. It is totally up to you when and how you fit these minutes into your daily routine.

But start now, and use these ideas to help make your workout part of the exercise.

Set a Smart Goal

A SMART purpose, according to ACE, is to be:

o   Specific

o   Measurable measurements

o   Achievable

o   Right

o   Time

Period (fulfilled with a deadline and completed in a specified period)

Having objectives helps to offer concentration and order to what you wish to do. Meeting targets is rewarding because it helps create excitement, exercise experts claim. Only pay particular attention to the portion of this equation that is "attainable."

Just an impossible target sets you up to struggle. Instead of forcing yourself to exercise for 30 minutes every day of the week because you can't even squeeze in 15 on other days, look at your calendar to find two days when you can raise your gym period to 30 minutes reasonably. All adds up to get you to your 150-minute week target.

Vowing to Take More Steps Each Day

For almost a decade, public health specialists at the CDC have encouraged Americans to take 10,000 steps per day. The 10,000 level averages out at around 5 miles a day, and "healthy" are known to be exercise far. Those that get in 12,500 steps a day are "very involved." Even if weight reduction is not your priority, you can improve your daily mileage to attain or sustain overall healthy health.

—

Render Exercise a Way of Life, Not a Fad

Some individuals make the error of going hard for exercise targets, but they slacken off after being reached. They use fitness as a means to a goal, not a way of living their lives. It will result in health conditions and weight gain. Failure to see health as a lifestyle option ensures that daily activity's long-term advantages would not be reaped.

Sure, in the short term, exercising will help you reduce or retain weight. Yet lifelong gains are created by an active lifestyle. It will lower the risk of future health problems, including:

· Elevated Blood Pressure
· Diabetes Nausea
· Cardiac Disorder
· Obesity

Exercise leads to better well-being and wellness, so make it a priority-it's never too late.

For Kidney Failure, What Foods Do You Eat?

It may be a little complicated at first to put together an excellent renal disease meal program, particularly if you don't know which foods you shouldn't eat with renal disease. People also want to think too deeply about what they cannot feed that they get overwhelmed to the extent that they don't know how much you can consume on a renal diet versus what you can eat. The trick is to reflect on the key ingredients you can avoid while still reflecting on the several choices that you do have available.

Here are a few explanations of kidney disorder foods that you can eat:

- **Foods Unprocessed**

In the U.S., in particular, people appear to rely on packaged foods to make their meals. Such goods are full of additives that are not safe for anybody, including an individual with renal disease. Vast quantities of salt and lots of other additives are loaded with packaged foods like canned cheese and macaroni meal helper sets and even plain rice dishes, which come in a package. As a familiar concept, you shouldn't consume anything if it arrives in a wooden box. It would help if you instead depended on natural foods to help the body regenerate and fill you up. When you're about to make any changes, learning what you should consume on a kidney diet helps. Without the additional preservatives, discover methods to make your preferred dishes from scratch.

- **The Natural Produce**

Sometimes, vegetables and fruit are considered natural medications for your health, so the produce department is always a perfect way to start while you search for groceries. It should always be in your cart or on your dining table, especially foods like bell peppers, onions, cabbage, and super-foods such as berries. Ensure that you're still paying care to your potassium consumption if you're in the latter stages of kidney disease, which may reduce your development choices a little more. You may ask what foods are produced not to consume with renal disease, but this depends on your process and diet limits. Check for more choices with our meal preparation solution: 21 Day Pre-Dialysis Kidney Disease Vegetarian Meal Schedule.

- **The Appropriate Grains**

Although your kidneys might not have processed some whole grain choices, you may always appreciate stuff like pasta and rice in moderation. To more straightforward, the kidneys absorb your consuming meal byproducts due to potassium & phosphorus limits, sticking to these ingredients' white varieties. You will appreciate the whole grain forms to raise fiber if you are not limited (Stage 3 / 4 CKD).

- **Spices and Herbs**

To make meals taste lovely, you do not need salt. If you sprinkle in numerous spices that are part of foods you may eat on a renal diet, you may begin to find that foods naturally taste more delightful and have deeper flavors than you have ever thought possible. Go for new or dried herbs & spices (salt-free) to season your meals anytime you need anything special to dress up the recipes.

- **Lean Proteins**

You might be or might not need to restrict the protein consumption, based on what process of renal disease you are in. However, it is recommended that most patients also serve lean protein at least once a day. Usually, fish, egg whites, poultry, and tofu are the top options. Fish is particularly useful for you, as it gives your diet with good healthy omega 3s. To create unique and satisfying meals, you can use any of these options, and the choices are as restricted as your imagination. Consider tacos, fajitas, casseroles, and much more, beginning with these excellent lean protein options.

You will start to create a tasty and balanced renal disease meal schedule, beginning with any of these food groups & examples. Before making a new diet, decisions, or changing what you consume for your renal illness, always consult a doctor.

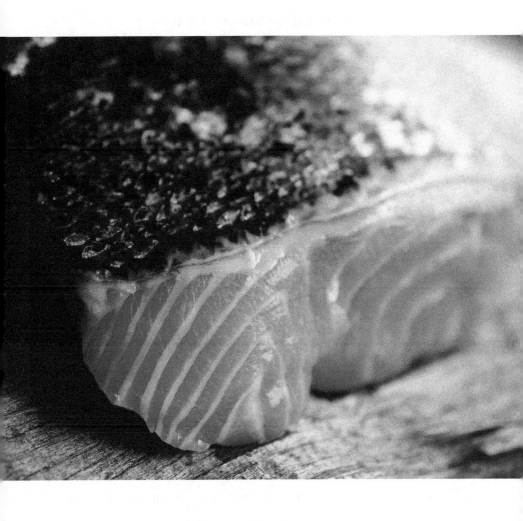

1. SHRIMP PAELLA

Preparation Time: 5 minutes

Cooking Time: 10 minutes

Servings: 2

Ingredients:

- 1 cup cooked brown rice
- 1 chopped red onion
- 1 teaspoon paprika
- 1 chopped garlic clove
- 1 tablespoon olive oil
- 6 oz. frozen cooked shrimp
- 1 deseeded and sliced chili pepper
- 1 tablespoon oregano

Directions:

1. Warm the olive oil in a pan on medium-high heat.
2. Add the onion and garlic and sauté for 2-3 minutes until soft.
3. Now add the shrimp and sauté for a further 5 minutes or until hot through.
4. Now add the herbs, spices, chili, and rice with 1/2 cup boiling water.

5. Stir until everything is warm and the water has been absorbed.

6. Plate up and serve.

Nutrition:

Calories 221,

Protein 17 g,

Carbohydrates 31 g,

Fat 8 g,

Sodium (Na) 235 mg,

Potassium (K) 176 mg,

Phosphorus 189 mg

2. Salmon and Pesto Salad

Preparation Time: 5 minutes

Cooking Time: 15 minutes

Servings: 2

Ingredients:

For the pesto:

- 1 minced garlic clove
- ½ cup fresh arugula
- ¼ cup extra virgin olive oil
- ½ cup fresh basil
- 1 teaspoon black pepper

For the salmon:

- 4 oz. skinless salmon fillet
- 1 tablespoon coconut oil

For the salad:

- ½ juiced lemon
- 2 sliced radishes
- ½ cup iceberg lettuce
- 1 teaspoon black pepper

Directions:

1. Prepare the pesto by blending all the fixings for the pesto in a food processor or by grinding with a pestle and mortar. Set aside.
2. Add a skillet to the stove on medium-high heat and melt the coconut oil.
3. Add the salmon to the pan.
4. Cook for 7-8 minutes and turn over.
5. Cook for an additional 3-4 minutes or pending cooked through.
6. Remove fillets from the skillet and allow to rest.
7. Mix the lettuce and the radishes and squeeze over the juice of ½ lemon.
8. Flake the salmon with a fork and mix through the salad.
9. Toss to coat and sprinkle with a little black pepper to serve.

Nutrition:

Calories 221,

Protein 13 g,

Carbohydrates 1 g,

Fat 34 g,

Sodium (Na) 80 mg,

Potassium (K) 119 mg,

Phosphorus 158 mg

3. BAKED FENNEL AND GARLIC SEA BASS

Preparation Time: 5 minutes

Cooking Time: 15 minutes

Servings: 2

Ingredients:

- 1 lemon
- ½ sliced fennel bulb
- 6 oz. sea bass fillets
- 1 teaspoon black pepper
- 2 garlic cloves

Directions:

1. Preheat the oven to 375°F
2. Sprinkle black pepper over the Sea Bass.
3. Slice the fennel bulb and garlic cloves.
4. Add 1 salmon fillet and half the fennel and garlic to one sheet of baking paper or tin foil.
5. Squeeze in 1/2 lemon juices.
6. Repeat for the other fillet.
7. Fold and add to the oven for 12-15 minutes or until fish is thoroughly cooked through.
8. Meanwhile, add boiling water to your couscous, cover, and allow to steam.
9. Serve with your choice of rice or salad.

Nutrition:

Calories 221,

Protein 14 g,

Carbohydrates 3 g,

Fat 2 g,

Sodium (Na) 119 mg,

Potassium (K) 398 mg,

Phosphorus 149 mg

4. LEMON, GARLIC & CILANTRO TUNA AND RICE

Preparation Time: 5 minutes

Cooking Time: 0 minutes

Servings: 2

Ingredients:

- ½ cup arugula
- 1 tablespoon extra-virgin olive oil
- 1 cup cooked rice
- 1 teaspoon black pepper
- ¼ finely diced red onion
- 1 juiced lemon
- 3 oz. canned tuna
- 2 tablespoons chopped fresh cilantro

Directions:

1. Mix the olive oil, pepper, cilantro, and red onion in a bowl.
2. Stir in the tuna, cover, and leave in the fridge for as long as possible (if you can). You may also serve it immediately.
3. When ready to eat, serve up with the cooked rice and arugula!

Nutrition:

Calories 221,

Protein 11 g,

Carbohydrates 26 g,

Fat 7 g,

Sodium (Na) 143 mg,

Potassium (K)197 mg,

Phosphorus 182 mg

5. Cod & Green Bean Risotto

Preparation Time: 4 minutes

Cooking Time: 40 minutes

Servings: 2

Ingredients:

- ½ cup arugula
- 1 finely diced white onion
- 4 oz. cod fillet
- 1 cup white rice
- 2 lemon wedges
- 1 cup boiling water
- ¼ teaspoon black pepper
- 1 cup low sodium chicken broth
- 1 tablespoon extra-virgin olive oil
- ½ cup green beans

Directions:

1. Heat the oil in a pot with medium heat.
2. Sauté the chopped onion for 5 minutes until soft before adding in the rice and stirring for 1-2 minutes.
3. Combine the broth with boiling water.
4. Add half of the liquid to the pan and stir slowly.
5. Slowly add the rest of the liquid whilst continuously stirring for up to 20-30 minutes.
6. Stir in the green beans to the risotto.

7. Place the fish on top of the rice, cover, and steam for 10 minutes.
8. Ensure the water does not dry out and keep topping up until the rice is cooked thoroughly.
9. Use your fork to break up the fish fillets and stir into the rice.
10. Sprinkle with freshly ground pepper and a squeeze of fresh lemon to serve.
11. Garnish with lemon wedges and serve with the arugula.

Nutrition:

Calories 221,

Protein 12 g,

Carbohydrates 29 g,

Fat 8 g,

Sodium (Na) 398 mg,

Potassium (K) 347 mg,

Phosphorus 241 mg

6. MIXED PEPPER STUFFED RIVER TROUT

Preparation Time: 5 minutes

Cooking Time: 20 minutes

Servings: 4

Ingredients:

- 1 whole river trout
- 1 teaspoon thyme
- ¼ diced yellow pepper
- 1 cup baby spinach leaves
- ¼ diced green pepper
- 1 juiced lime
- ¼ diced red pepper
- 1 teaspoon oregano
- 1 teaspoon extra virgin olive oil
- 1 teaspoon black pepper

Directions:

1. Preheat the broiler /grill on high heat.
2. Lightly oil a baking tray.
3. Mix all the ingredients apart from the trout and lime.
4. Slice the trout lengthways (there should be an opening here from where it was gutted) and stuff the mixed ingredients inside.
5. Squeeze the lime juice over the fish and then place the lime wedges on the tray.

6. Place under the broiler on the baking tray and broil for 15-20 minutes or until fish is thoroughly cooked through and flakes easily.

7. Enjoy the dish as it is, or with a side helping of rice or salad.

Nutrition:

Calories 290,

Protein 15 g,

Carbohydrates 0 g,

Fat 7 g,

Sodium (Na) 43 mg,

Potassium (K) 315 mg,

Phosphorus 189 mg

7. HADDOCK & BUTTERED LEEKS

Preparation Time: 5 minutes

Cooking Time: 15 minutes

Servings: 2

Ingredients:

- 1 tablespoon unsalted butter
- 1 sliced leek
- ¼ teaspoon black pepper

- 2 teaspoons chopped parsley
- 6 oz. haddock fillets
- ½ juiced lemon

Directions:

1. Preheat the oven to 375°F
2. Add the haddock fillets to baking or parchment paper and sprinkle with the black pepper.
3. Squeeze over the lemon juice and wrap into a parcel.
4. Bake the parcel on a baking tray for 10-15 minutes or until the fish is thoroughly cooked through.
5. Meanwhile, heat the butter over medium-low heat in a small pan.
6. Add the leeks and parsley and sauté for 5-7 minutes until soft.
7. Serve the haddock fillets on a bed of buttered leeks and enjoy!

Nutrition:

Calories 124,

Protein 15 g,

Carbohydrates 0 g,

Fat 7 g,

Sodium (Na) 161 mg,

Potassium (K) 251 mg,

Phosphorus 220 mg

8. THAI SPICED HALIBUT

Preparation Time: 5 minutes

Cooking Time: 20 minutes

Servings: 2

Ingredients:

- 2 tablespoons coconut oil
- 1 cup white rice
- ¼ teaspoon black pepper
- ½ diced red chili
- 1 tablespoon fresh basil
- 2 pressed garlic cloves
- 4 oz. halibut fillet
- 1 halved lime
- 2 sliced green onions
- 1 lime leaf

Directions:

1. Preheat oven to 400°F/Gas Mark 5.
2. Add half of the ingredients into baking paper and fold into a parcel.
3. Repeat for your second parcel.
4. Add to the oven for 15-20 minutes or until fish is thoroughly cooked through.
5. Serve with cooked rice.

Nutrition:

Calories 311,

Protein 16 g,

Carbohydrates 17 g,

Fat 15 g,

Sodium (Na) 31 mg,

Potassium (K) 418 mg,

Phosphorus 257 mg

9. Homemade Tuna Niçoise

Preparation Time: 5 minutes

Cooking Time: 10 minutes

Servings: 2

Ingredients:

- 1 egg
- ½ cup green beans
- ¼ sliced cucumber
- 1 juiced lemon
- 1 teaspoon black pepper
- ¼ sliced red onion
- 1 tablespoon olive oil
- 1 tablespoon capers
- 4 oz. drained canned tuna
- 4 iceberg lettuce leaves
- 1 teaspoon chopped fresh cilantro

Directions:

1. Prepare the salad by washing and slicing the lettuce, cucumber, and onion.
2. Add to a salad bowl.
3. Mix 1 tablespoon oil with lemon juice, cilantro, and capers for a salad dressing. Set aside.

4. Boil a pan of water on high heat, then lower to simmer and add the egg for 6 minutes. (Steam the green beans over the same pan in a steamer/colander for 6 minutes).

5. Remove the egg and rinse under cold water.

6. Peel before slicing in half.

7. Mix the tuna, salad, and dressing together in a salad bowl.

8. Toss to coat.

9. Top with the egg and serve with a sprinkle of black pepper.

Nutrition:

Calories 199,

Protein 19 g,

Carbohydrates 7 g,

Fat 8 g,

Sodium (Na) 466 mg,

Potassium (K) 251 mg,

Phosphorus 211 mg

10. MONK-FISH CURRY

Preparation Time: 5 minutes

Cooking Time: 20 minutes

Servings: 2

Ingredients:

- 1 garlic clove
- 3 finely chopped green onions
- 1 teaspoon grated ginger
- 1 cup of water.
- 2 teaspoons chopped fresh basil
- 1 cup cooked rice noodles
- 1 tablespoon coconut oil
- ½ sliced red chili
- 4 oz. Monkfish fillet
- ½ finely sliced stick lemongrass
- 2 tablespoons chopped shallots

Directions:

1. Slice the Monkfish into bite-size pieces.
2. Using mortar and pestle or food processor, crush the basil, garlic, ginger, chili, and lemongrass to form a paste.
3. Heat the oil in a large wok or pan over medium-high heat and add the shallots.

4. Now add the water to the pan and bring to a boil.

5. Add the Monkfish, lower the heat, and cover to simmer for 10 minutes or until cooked through.

6. Enjoy with rice noodles and scatter with green onions to serve.

Nutrition:

Calories 249,

Protein 12 g,

Carbohydrates 30 g,

Fat 10 g,

Sodium (Na) 32 mg,

Potassium (K) 398 mg,

Phosphorus 190 mg

11. Oregon Tuna Patties

Preparation Time: 10 minutes

Cooking Time: 15 minutes

Servings: 4

Ingredients:

- 1 (14.75 ounces) can of tuna

- 2 tablespoons butter

- 1 medium onion, chopped

- 2/3 cup graham cracker crumbs

- 2 egg whites, beaten

- 1/4 cup chopped fresh parsley

- 1 teaspoon dry mustard

- 3 tablespoons olive oil

Directions:

1. Drain the tuna, reserving 3/4 cup of the liquid. Flake the meat. Thaw butter in a large skillet over medium-high heat. Add onion, and cook until tender.

2. In a medium bowl, combine the onions with the reserved tuna liquid, 1/3 of the graham cracker crumbs, egg whites, parsley, mustard, and tuna. Mix until well blended, then shape into six patties. Coat patties in remaining cracker crumbs.

3. Heat olive in a large skillet over medium heat. Cook patties until browned, then carefully turn and brown on the other side.

Nutrition:

Calories 204,

Total Fat 15.4g,

Saturated Fat 4.4g,

Cholesterol 74mg,

Sodium 111mg,

Total Carbohydrate 6.5g,

Dietary Fiber 0.9g,

Total Sugar 2g,

Protein 10.5g,

Calcium 21mg,

Iron 1mg,

Potassium 164mg,

Phosphorus 106mg

12. FISH CHOWDER

Preparation Time: 20 minutes

Cooking Time: 40 minutes

Servings: 4

Ingredients:

- 2 tablespoons butter

- 2 cups chopped onion

- 4 fresh mushrooms, sliced

- 1 stalk celery, chopped

- 4 cups chicken stock

- 2 pounds' cod, diced into 1/2-inch cubes

- 1/2 cup all-purpose flour

- 1/8 teaspoon Mrs. Dash salt-free seasoning, or to taste

- Ground black pepper to taste

- 2 (12 fluid ounce) cans soy milk

Directions:

1. In a large stockpot, melt two tablespoons of butter over medium heat. Sauté onions, mushrooms, and celery in butter until tender.

2. Add chicken stock simmer for 10 minutes.

3. Add cod, and simmer another 10 minutes.

4. Mix flour until smooth; stir into soup and simmer for 1 minute more. Season to taste with seasoning and pepper. Remove from heat, and stir in soy milk.

Nutrition:

Calories 171,

Total Fat 4.2g,

Saturated Fat 2.1g,

Cholesterol 32mg,

Sodium 810mg,

Total Carbohydrate 19.3g,

Dietary Fiber 2g,

Total Sugar 3.9g,

Protein 14.1g,

Calcium 41mg,

Iron 2mg,

Potassium 204mg,

Phosphorus 106mg

13. Broiled Sesame Cod

Preparation Time: 5 minutes

Cooking Time: 10 minutes

Servings: 4

Ingredients:

- 1/2 pounds' cod fillets

- 1 teaspoon butter, melted

- 1 teaspoon lemon juice

- 1 teaspoon dried basil

- 1 pinch ground black pepper

- 1 tablespoon sesame seeds

Directions:

1. Preheat the oven's broiler then set the oven rack approximately 6 inches from the heat source.

2. Place the cod fillets on the foil, and brush with butter. Season it using lemon juice, basil, and black pepper; sprinkle with sesame seeds.

3. Broil the fish in the warmed broiler until the flesh turns opaque and white, and the fish flakes easily, about 10 minutes.

Nutrition:

Calories 67,

Total Fat 2.6g,

Saturated Fat 0.8g,

Cholesterol 30mg,

Sodium 43mg,

Total Carbohydrate 0.6g,

Dietary Fiber 0.3g,

Total Sugar 0g,

Protein 10.6g,

Calcium 23mg,

Iron 0mg,

Potassium 13mg,

Phosphorus 10mg

14. TUNA SALAD WITH CRANBERRIES

Preparation Time: 10 minutes

Cooking Time: 0 minutes

Servings: 4

Ingredient:

- 2 (5 ounces) cans of solid white tuna
- 2 tablespoons mayonnaise
- 1/3 teaspoon dried dill weed
- 3 tablespoons dried cranberries

Directions:

1. Put the tuna in a bowl, and puree with a fork.

2. Put in mayonnaise to evenly coat tuna. Mix in dill and cranberries.

3. Enjoy on crackers or the bread of your choice!

Nutrition:

Calories 81,

Total Fat 2.8g,

Saturated Fat 0.5g,

Cholesterol 15mg,

Sodium 74mg,

Total Carbohydrate 2.3g,

Dietary Fiber 0.2g,

Total Sugar 0.7g,

Protein 10.9g,

Calcium 8mg,

Iron 1mg,

Potassium 113mg,

Phosphorus 95mg

15. ZUCCHINI CUPS WITH DILL CREAM AND SMOKED TUNA

Preparation Time: 15 minutes

Cooking Time: 35 minutes

Servings: 4

Ingredients:

- 1 1/3 large Zucchini
- 4 ounces' cream cheese, softened
- 2 tablespoons chopped fresh dill

- 1 teaspoon lemon zest

- 1/2 teaspoon fresh lemon juice

- 1/4 teaspoon ground black pepper

- 4 ounces smoked tuna, cut into 2-inch strips

Directions:

1. Trim ends from Zucchini and cut crosswise into 24 rounds. Scoop a 1/2-inch-deep depression from one side of each round with a small melon-baller, forming little cups. Drain Zucchini, cup sides down, on paper towels for 15 minutes.

2. Beat cream cheese, chopped dill, lemon zest, lemon juice, and black pepper together in a bowl.

3. The next thing you will do is to spoon 1/2 teaspoon cheese mixture into each Zucchini cup. Then top each cup with one tuna strip.

Nutrition:

Calories 51,

Total Fat 3.8g,

Saturated Fat 2.2g,

Cholesterol 13mg,

Sodium 219mg,

Total Carbohydrate 1.8g,

Dietary Fiber 0.3g,

Total Sugar 0.6g,

Protein 2.8g,

Calcium 24mg,

Iron 1mg,

Potassium 95mg,

Phosphorus 40mg

16. CREAMY SMOKED TUNA MACARONI

Preparation Time: 15 minutes

Cooking Time: 25 minutes

Servings: 4

Ingredients:

- 3 tablespoons olive oil
- ¼ onion, finely chopped
- 1 tablespoon all-purpose flour
- 1 teaspoon garlic powder

- 1 cup of soy milk

- ¼ cup cream cheese

- ½ cup frozen green peas, thawed and drained

- ¼ cup canned mushrooms, drained

- 5 ounces smoked tuna, chopped

- ½ (16 ounces) package macaroni

Directions:

1. Boil a large pot of water. Put the macaroni and cook for 8 to 10 minutes or until al dente; drain.
2. Heat oil in a large skillet over medium heat. Sauté onion in oil until tender.
3. Stir flour and garlic powder into the oil and onions. Gradually stir in milk. Heat to just a lower boiling point, and then slowly stir in cheese until the sauce is smooth. Stir in peas and mushrooms. And cook over low heat for 4 minutes.
4. Toss in smoked tuna, and cook for two more minutes. Serve over macaroni.

Nutrition:

Calories 147,

Total Fat 8.3g,

Saturated Fat 1.9g,

Cholesterol 14mg,

Sodium 979mg,

Total Carbohydrate 6.5g,

Dietary Fiber 0.8g,

Total Sugar 1.9g,

Protein 11.4g,

Calcium 38mg,

Iron 1mg,

Potassium 160mg,

Phosphorus 100mg

17. Asparagus and Smoked Tuna Salad

Preparation Time: 15 minutes

Cooking Time: 10 minutes

Servings: 4

Ingredients:

- ½ pound fresh asparagus
- 1 heads lettuce, rinsed and torn
- ¼ cup frozen green peas, thawed
- 1/8 cup olive oil
- 1 tablespoon lemon juice
- ½ teaspoon Dijon mustard
- 1/8 teaspoon pepper
- 1/8-pound smoked tuna, cut into 1inch chunks

Directions:

1. Boil a pot of water. Put the asparagus in the pot, and cook 5 minutes, just until tender. Drain, and set aside.
2. In a large bowl, toss the asparagus, lettuce, peas, and tuna.
3. In a separate bowl, mix the olive oil, lemon juice, Dijon mustard, and pepper. Put it with the salad or serve on the side.

Nutrition:

Calories 87,

Total Fat 7g,

Saturated Fat 1.1g,

Cholesterol 3mg,

Sodium 298mg,

Total Carbohydrate 2.7g,

Dietary Fiber 1.1g,

Total Sugar 1g,

Protein 3.8g,

Calcium 16mg,

Iron 1mg,

Potassium 134mg,

Phosphorus 104 mg

18. Spicy Tuna Salad Sandwiches

Preparation Time: 15 minutes

Cooking Time: 0 minutes

Servings: 2

Ingredient:

- 1 (8 ounces) can tuna, undrained
- 1/4 cucumber, chopped
- 2 tablespoons light mayonnaise
- 1 tablespoon vinegar
- 1 teaspoon red chili paste
- 4 slices white bread, toasted

Directions:

1. Put tuna into a bowl and use a fork to flake and mix with the liquid from the can.
2. Mix cucumber with the tuna.
3. Stir mayonnaise, vinegar, chili paste together in a bowl; add hot sauce and adjust to taste.
4. Pour mayonnaise mixture over the salmon mixture and stir to coat.
5. Spoon onto toasted bread to make sandwiches.

Nutrition:

Calories 189,

Total Fat 7.6g,

Saturated Fat 1.1g,

Cholesterol 28mg,

Sodium 326mg,

Total Carbohydrate 15.6g,

Dietary Fiber 2.1g,

Total Sugar 3.4g,

Protein 15.1g,

Calcium 60mg,

Iron 1mg,

Potassium 119mg,

Phosphorus 109 mg

19. Spanish Tuna

Preparation Time: 20 minutes

Cooking Time: 15 minutes

Servings: 4

Ingredients:

- 1 tablespoon olive oil

- 1/4 cup finely chopped onion

- 2 tablespoons chopped fresh garlic

- 1/4 cup basil chopped

- 1 dash black pepper

- 1 dash cayenne pepper

- 1 dash paprika

- 6 (4 ounce) fillets tuna fillets

Directions:

1. Warm olive oil in a pan with medium heat.

2. Cook and stir onions and garlic until onions are slightly tender; careful not to burn the garlic.

3. Season with black pepper, cayenne pepper, basil, and paprika.

4. Cook fillets in sauce over medium heat for 5 to 8 minutes, or until easily flaked with a fork. Serve immediately.

Nutrition:

Calories 130,

Total Fat 4.6g,

Saturated Fat 0.5g,

Cholesterol 55mg,

Sodium 71mg,

Total Carbohydrate 2.2g,

Dietary Fiber 0.3g,

Total Sugar 0.4g,

Protein 20.4g,

Calcium 10mg,

Iron 0mg,

Potassium 31mg,

Phosphorus 46 mg

20. FISH WITH VEGETABLES

Preparation Time: 30 minutes

Cooking Time: 60 minutes

Servings: 4

Ingredients:

- 1 egg white, beaten

- ¼ cup all-purpose flour

- Black pepper to taste

- 1-pound firm salmon fillets, cut into 1 1/2-inch piece

- ½ cup olive oil, divided

- 1 onion, cut in half, and thinly sliced

- 1 carrot, peeled and coarsely grated

- ½ large turnips, peeled and coarsely grated

- 1/2 leek coarsely grated

- 1 cup of water

Directions:

1. Place egg white and flour in 2 shallow bowls. Season egg white with pepper.

2. Dip fish pieces first in the beaten egg, then dredge in the flour.

3. Warm 1/4 cup olive oil in a deep-frying pan with medium heat until hot.

4. Add fish in batches and fry on both sides until golden, 5 to 8 minutes per batch.

5. Take away fish from skillet and set aside.

6. Heat remaining 1/4 cup oil in a distinct skillet and cook onions until soft and translucent, about 5 minutes. Add carrots, turnips, and leek; mix well.

7. Add water and season with pepper. Close the lid and simmer on low heat until vegetables are soft about 30 minutes.

8. Check and add more water if the mixture becomes too dry.

9. Arrange vegetables and fried fish in a 10-inch round serving dish, starting and ending with vegetables.

Nutrition:

Calories 358,

Total Fat 30.1g,

Saturated Fat 6g,

Cholesterol 57mg,

Sodium 45mg,

Total Carbohydrate 14.7g,

Dietary Fiber 2.2g,

Total Sugar 3.3g,

Protein 8.2g,

Calcium 38mg,

Iron 1mg,

Potassium 281mg,

Phosphorus 161 mg

21. CREAMY CRAB OVER SALMON

Preparation Time: 10 minutes

Cooking Time: 15 minutes

Servings: 4

Ingredients:

- 1/4 cup olive oil, divided
- 2 (4 ounces) fillets of salmon
- 1 teaspoon dried oregano
- 1 pinch ground white pepper
- 1 3/4 cups soy milk
- 4 ounces' fresh crabmeat
- 1 teaspoon lemon juice

Directions:

1. Heat a small amount of olive oil in a non-stick skillet over medium heat.
2. Season salmon with oregano and white pepper; cook in skillet until the flesh flakes easily with a fork, 7 to 10 minutes per side.
3. While fish cooks, whisk remaining olive oil, soy milk together in a saucepan over medium-low heat; cook, stirring regularly, until it begins to thicken, 3 to 5 minutes.
4. Remove saucepan from heat and stir crab meat into the sauce.

5. Transfer cooked cod to plates and spoon sauce over the fish.

Nutrition:

Calories 258,

Total Fat 16.5g,

Saturated Fat 2.5g,

Cholesterol 40mg,

Sodium 395mg,

Total Carbohydrate 11.4g,

Dietary Fiber 1g,

Total Sugar 6.1g,

Protein 17.3g,

Calcium 37mg,

Iron 1mg,

Potassium 160mg,

Potassium 120mg

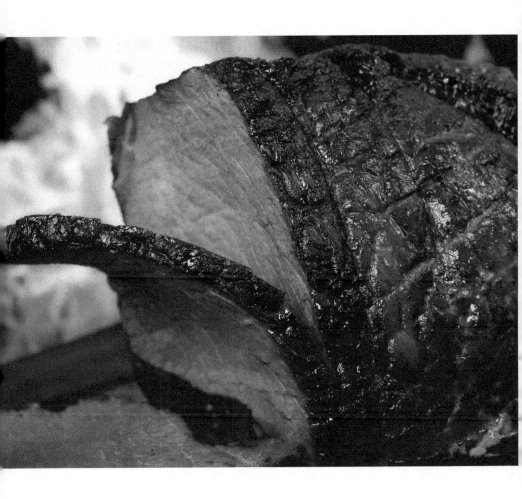

22. SLOW-COOKED BEEF BRISKET

Preparation Time: 10 minutes

Cooking Time: 3 hours and 30 minutes

Servings: 6

Ingredients:

- 10-ounce chuck roast
- 1 onion, sliced
- 1 cup carrots, peeled and sliced
- 1 tablespoon mustard
- 1 tablespoon thyme (fresh or dried)
- 1 tablespoon rosemary (fresh or dried)
- 2 garlic cloves
- 2 tablespoons extra-virgin olive oil
- 1 teaspoon black pepper
- 1 cup homemade chicken stock (p.52)
- 1 cup of water

Directions:

1. Preheat oven to 300F

2. Trim any fat from the beef and soak vegetables in warm water.

3. Make a paste by mixing the mustard, thyme, rosemary, and garlic, before mixing in the oil and pepper.

4. Combine this mix with the stock.

5. Pour the mixture over the beef into an ovenproof baking dish.

6. Place the vegetables onto the bottom of the baking dish with the beef.

7. Cover and roast for 3 hours, or until tender.

8. Uncover the dish then continue to cook for 30 minutes in the oven.

9. Serve hot!

Nutrition:

Calories: 151

Fat: 7g

Carbohydrates: 7g

Phosphorus: 144mg

Potassium: 344mg:

Sodium: 279mg

Protein: 15g

23. PORK SOUVLAKI

Preparation time: 20 minutes

Cooking time: 12 minutes

Servings: 8

Ingredients:

- Olive oil – 3 tablespoons
- Lemon juice – 2 tablespoons
- Minced garlic – 1 teaspoon
- Chopped fresh oregano – 1 tablespoon
- Ground black pepper – ¼ teaspoon
- Pork leg – 1 pound, cut into 2-inch cubes

Directions:

1. In a bowl, stir together the lemon juice, olive oil, garlic, oregano, and pepper.

2. Add the pork cubes and toss to coat.

3. Place the bowl in the refrigerator, covered, for 2 hours to marinate.

4. Thread the pork chunks onto eight wooden skewers that have been soaked in water.

5. Preheat the barbecue to medium-high heat.

6. Grill the pork skewers for about 12 minutes, turning once, until just cooked through but still juicy.

Nutrition:

Calories: 95

Fat: 4g Carb: 0g

Phosphorus: 125mg

Potassium: 230mg

Sodium: 29mg

Protein: 13g

24. Open-Faced Beef Stir-Up

Preparation time: 10 minutes

Cooking time: 10 minutes

Servings: 6

Ingredients:

- 95% Lean ground beef – ½ pound
- Chopped sweet onion – ½ cup
- Shredded cabbage – ½ cup
- Herb pesto – ¼ cup
- Hamburger buns – 6, bottom halves only

Directions:

1. Sauté the beef and onion for 6 minutes or until beef is cooked.

2. Add the cabbage and sauté for 3 minutes more.

3. Stir in pesto and heat for 1 minute.

4. Divide the beef mixture into six portions and serve each on the bottom half of a hamburger bun, open-face.

Nutrition:

Calories: 120

Fat: 3g

Phosphorus: 106mg

Potassium: 198mg

Sodium: 134mg

Protein: 11g

25. Grilled Steak with Cucumber Salsa

Preparation time: 20 minutes

Cooking time: 15 minutes

Servings: 4

Ingredients:

For the salsa:

- Boiled and diced red bell pepper – ¼ cup
- Chopped English cucumber – 1 cup
- Scallion – 1, both green and white parts, chopped
- Chopped fresh cilantro – 2 tablespoons
- Juice of 1 lime

For the steak:

- Olive oil
- Beef tenderloin steaks – 4(3-ounce), room temperature
- Freshly ground black pepper

Directions:

1. In a bowl, to make the salsa combine the lime juice, cilantro, scallion, bell pepper, and cucumber. Set aside.

2. To make the steak: Preheat a barbecue to medium heat.

3. Rub the steaks all over with oil and season with pepper.

4. Grill the steaks for about 5 minutes per side for medium-rare, or until the desired state.

5. Serve the steaks topped with salsa.

Nutrition:

Calories: 130

Fat: 6g

Carb: 1g

Phosphorus: 186mg

Potassium: 272mg

Sodium: 39mg

Protein: 19g

26. BEEF BRISKET

Preparation time: 10 minutes

Cooking time: 3 ½ hours

Servings: 6

Ingredients:

- Chuck roast – 12 ounces trimmed
  - Garlic – 2 cloves
  - Thyme – 1 tablespoon
  - Rosemary – tablespoon
  - Mustard - 1 tablespoon
  - Extra virgin olive oil – ¼ cup
  - Black pepper – 1 teaspoon
  - Onion – 1, diced
  - Carrots – 1 cup, peeled and sliced
  - Low salt stock – 2 cups

Directions:

1. Preheat the oven to 300F.

2. Soak vegetables in warm water.

3. Make a paste by mixing the thyme, mustard, rosemary, and garlic. Then mix in the oil and pepper.

4. Add the beef to the dish.

5. Pour the mixture over the beef into a dish.

6. Place the vegetables onto the bottom of the baking dish around the beef.

7. Cover and roast for 3 hours, or until tender.

8. Uncover the dish then continue to cook for 30 minutes in the oven.

9. Serve.

Nutrition:

Calories: 303

Fat: 25g

Carb: 7g

Phosphorus: 376mg

Potassium: 246mg

Sodium: 44mg

Protein: 18g

27. Apricot and Lamb Tagine

Preparation time: 10 minutes

Cooking time: 1 to 1 ½ hour

Servings: 2

Ingredients:

- Extra virgin olive oil – 1 tablespoon
- Lean lamb fillets – 2, cubed
- Onion – 1, diced
- Homemade chicken stock – 4 cups
- Cumin – 1 teaspoon
- Turmeric – 1 teaspoon
- Curry powder – 1 teaspoon
- Dried rosemary – 1 teaspoon
- Chopped parsley – 1 teaspoon
- Canned apricots – ½ cup, juices drained, and apricots rinsed

Directions:

1. Heat the olive oil in a pot.

2. Add lamb to the pot and cook for 5 minutes or until browned.

3. Remove lamb and set aside.

4. Add the chopped onion to the pot and sauté for 5 minutes, or until starting to soften.

5. Sprinkle with cumin, curry powder, and turmeric over the onions and continue to stir for 4 to 5 minutes.

6. Now put the lamb again into the pot with the chicken stock and rosemary.

7. Cover the pot and leave to simmer on low heat for 1 to 1.5 hours or until the lamb is tender and fully cooked through.

8. Add the apricots 15 minutes before the end of the cooking time.

9. Garnish with parsley and serve.

Nutrition:

Calories: 193

Fat: 12g

Carb: 9g

Phosphorus: 170mg

Potassium: 156mg

Sodium: 105mg

Protein: 20g

28. Lamb Shoulder with Zucchini and Eggplant

Preparation time: 10 minutes

Cooking time: 4 to 5 hours

Servings: 2

Ingredients:

- Lean lamb shoulder – 6 ounces
- Zucchinis – 2, cubed
- Eggplant – 1, cubed
- Black pepper – 1 teaspoon
- Extra virgin olive oil – 2 tablespoons
- Basil – 1 tablespoon
- Oregano – 1 tablespoon
- Garlic – 2 cloves, chopped

Directions:

1. Preheat the oven to its highest setting.

2. Soak the vegetables in warm water.

3. Trim any fat from the lamb shoulder.

4. Rub the lamb with one tablespoon of olive oil, pepper, and herbs.

5. Line a baking tray with the rest of the olive oil, garlic, zucchini, and eggplant.

6. Add the lamb shoulder and cover with foil.

7. Turn the oven down to 325F and add the dish into the oven.

8. Cook for 4 to 5 hours, remove and rest.

9. Slice the lamb then serve with the vegetables.

Nutrition:

Calories: 478

Fat: 31g

Carb: 13g

Phosphorus: 197mg

Potassium: 414mg

Sodium: 84mg

Protein: 33g

29. Beef Chili

Preparation time: 10 minutes

Cooking time: 30 minutes

Servings: 2

Ingredients:

- Onion – 1, diced
- Red bell pepper – 1, diced
- Garlic – 2 cloves, minced
- Lean ground beef – 6 ounces
- Chili powder – 1 teaspoon
- Oregano – 1 teaspoon
- Extra virgin olive oil – 2 tablespoons
- Water – 1 cup
- Brown rice -1 cup
- Fresh cilantro – 1 tablespoon, to serve

Directions:

1. Soak vegetables in warm water.

2. Boil a pan of water then add rice for 20 minutes.

3. Meanwhile, add the oil to a pan and heat on medium-high heat.

4. Add the pepper, onions, and garlic and sauté for 5 minutes until soft.

5. Remove and set aside.

6. Add the beef to the pan and stir until browned.

7. Add the vegetables again into the pan and stir.

8. Now add the chili powder and herbs and water, cover, and turn the heat down a little to simmer for 15 minutes.

9. Meanwhile, drain the rice and add the lid, and steam while the chili is cooking.

10. Serve hot with the fresh cilantro sprinkled over the top.

Nutrition:

Calories: 459

Fat: 22g

Carb: 36g

Phosphorus: 332mg

Potassium: 360mg

Protein: 22g

30. Skirt Steak Glazed with Bourbon

Preparation Time: 30 minutes

Cooking Time: 50 minutes (1 hour additional)

Servings: 8

Ingredients:

Bourbon Glaze

- Shallots (diced) – ¼ cup
- Unsalted butter (chilled) – 3 tablespoons
- Bourbon – 1 cup
- Dark brown sugar – ¼ cup
- Dijon mustard – 2 tablespoons
- Black pepper – 1 tablespoon

Skirt Steak

- Grapeseed oil – 2 tablespoons
- Dried oregano – ½ teaspoon
- Smoked paprika – ½ teaspoon
- Black pepper – 1 teaspoon
- Red wine vinegar – 1 tablespoon
- Skirt steak – 2 pounds

Directions:

1. Start by preparing the bourbon glaze. For this, you will need to take a small saucepan and place it over a medium-high flame.

2. Add in 1 tablespoon of butter and toss in the shallots. Stir-fry until they turn brown.

3. Reduce the heat to the minimum and remove the saucepan from the stove. Pour in the bourbon and stir thoroughly. Return the saucepan to the stove.

4. Let this cook on a low flame for around 15 minutes. Make sure the glaze reduces to one-third.

5. Stir in the dark sugar, black pepper, and Dijon mustard. Keep stirring until the glaze becomes bubbly.

6. Turn off the flame and add in about two tablespoons of cold butter. Keep stirring to incorporate with the sauce.

7. Now prepare the skirt steak. To do this, take a gallon-sized zip-lock bag and add in the grapeseed oil, dried oregano, smoked paprika, black pepper, and red wine vinegar. Mix well.

8. Now add in the steaks and shake well. Allow the steaks to sit in the marinade for about 45 minutes.

9. Remove the steaks from the zip-lock bag. Set aside.

10. Heat the grill and place the steaks on it. Cook for about 20 minutes.

11. Once done, remove the steak and place it on a baking tray. Let it rest for about 10 minutes before serving.

12. Slice the steaks and drizzle the glaze on top. Place the tray in the broiler for 5 minutes. Serve hot!

Nutrition:

Protein 24 g

Carbohydrates 8 g

Fat 22 g

Cholesterol 93 mg

Sodium 152 mg

Potassium 283 mg

Phosphorus 171 mg

Calcium 22 mg

Fiber 0.5 g

31. BEEF POT ROAST

Preparation Time: 20 minutes

Cooking Time: 1 hour

Servings: 3

Ingredients:

- Round bone roast

- 2 - 4 pounds' chuck roast

Directions:

1. Trim off excess fat.
2. Pour a tablespoon of oil into a pan and heat to medium.
3. Roll pot roast in flour and brown on all sides in a hot skillet.
4. After the meat gets a brown color, reduce heat to low.
5. Season with pepper and herbs and add ½ cup of water.
6. Cook slowly for 1½ hours or until it looks ready.

Nutrition:

Calories 157

Protein 24 g

Fat 13 g

Carbs 0 g

Phosphorus 204 mg

Sodium (Na) 50 mg

32. GRILLED LAMB CHOPS

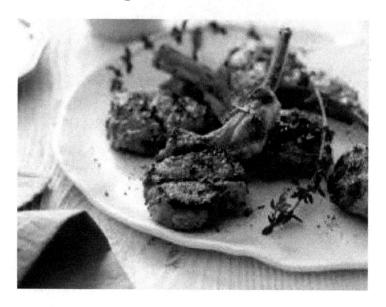

Preparation Time: 10 minutes

Cooking Time: 6 minutes

Serving: 1

Ingredients:

- 1 tablespoon fresh ginger, grated

- 4 garlic cloves, chopped roughly

- 1 teaspoon ground cumin

- ½ teaspoon red chili powder

- Salt and freshly ground black pepper

- 1 tablespoon essential olive oil

- 1 tablespoon fresh lemon juice

- 8 lamb chops, trimmed

Directions:

1. In a bowl, mix all fixings except chops.

2. With a hand blender, blend till a smooth mixture is formed.

3. Add chops and coat generously with mixture.

4. Refrigerate to marinate overnight.

5. Preheat the barbecue grill till hot. Grease the grill grate.

6. Grill the chops for approximately 3 minutes per side.

7. Serve when done.

Nutrition:

Calories: 227;

Fat: 12g;

Phosphorus: 36mg;

Potassium: 194mg;

Sodium: 31mg;

Carbohydrates: 1g;

Fiber: 0g;

Protein: 30g.

33. Lamb & Pineapple Kebabs

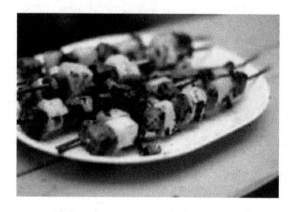

Preparation Time: 15 minutes

Cooking Time: 10 minutes

Serving: 1

Ingredients:

- 1 large pineapple, cubed into 1½-inch size, divided
- 1 (½-inch) piece fresh ginger, chopped
- 2 garlic cloves, chopped
- Salt, to taste
- 16-24-ounce lamb shoulder steak, trimmed and cubed into 1½-inch size
- Fresh mint leaves coming from a bunch
- The ground cinnamon, to taste

Directions:

1. Add about one half of pineapple, ginger, garlic, and salt and pulse till smooth in a blender.

2. Transfer the mixture into a large bowl.

3. Add chops and coat generously with the mixture.

4. Refrigerate to marinate for about 1-2 hours.

5. Preheat the grill to medium heat. Grease the grill grate.

6. Thread lam, remaining pineapple, and mint leaves onto pre-soaked wooden skewers.

7. Grill the kebabs for approximately 10 minutes, turning occasionally.

8. Serve when done.

Nutrition:

Calories: 482;

Fat: 16g;

Phosphorus: 36mg;

Potassium: 194mg;

Sodium: 31mg;

Carbohydrates: 22g;

Fiber: 5g;

Protein: 377g.

34. BAKED MEATBALLS & SCALLIONS

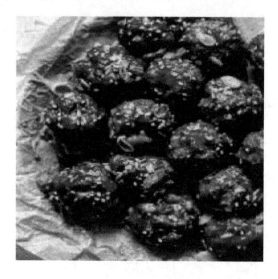

Preparation Time: 20 minutes

Cooking Time: 35 minutes

Serving: 1

Ingredients:

For Meatballs:

- 1 lemongrass stalk, outer skin peeled and chopped

- 1 (1½-inch) piece fresh ginger, sliced

- 3 garlic cloves, chopped

- 1 cup fresh cilantro leaves, chopped roughly

- ½ cup fresh basil leaves, chopped roughly

- 2 tablespoons plus 1 teaspoon fish sauce

- 2 tablespoons water

- 2 tablespoons fresh lime juice

- ½ pound lean ground pork

- 1-pound lean ground lamb

- 1 carrot, peeled and grated

- 1 organic egg, beaten

For Scallions:

- 16 stalks scallions, trimmed

- 2 tablespoons coconut oil, melted

- Salt, to taste

- ½ cup of water

Directions:

1. Preheat the oven to 3750 F. Grease a baking dish.

2. In a blender, add lemongrass, ginger, garlic, fresh herbs, fish sauce, water, and lime juice and pulse till chopped finely.

3. Transfer the mixture to a bowl with the remaining ingredients and mix well.

4. Make about 1-inch balls from the mixture.

5. Arrange the balls into the prepared baking dish in a single layer.

6. In another rimmed baking dish, arrange scallion stalks in a single layer.

7. Drizzle with coconut oil and sprinkle with salt.

8. Pour water into the baking dish, then, with foil paper, cover it tightly.

9. Bake the scallion for around a half-hour.

10. Bake the meatballs for approximately 30-35 minutes.

11. Serve the meatballs and scallion when done.

Nutrition:

Calories: 432;

Fat: 13g;

Phosphorus: 45mg;

Potassium: 78mg;

Sodium: 34mg;

Carbohydrates: 25g;

Fiber: 8g;

Protein: 40g.

35. PORK WITH BELL PEPPER

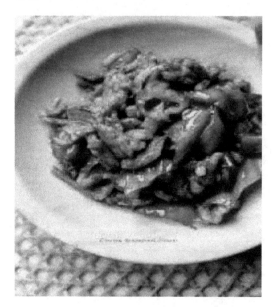

Preparation Time: 15 minutes

Cooking Time: 13 minutes

Serving: 1

Ingredients:

- 1 tablespoon fresh ginger, chopped finely

- 4 garlic cloves, chopped finely

- 1 cup fresh cilantro, chopped and divided

- ¼ cup plus 1 tablespoon olive oil, divided

- 1-pound tender pork, trimmed, sliced thinly

- 2 onions,

- 1 green bell pepper

- 1 tablespoon fresh lime juice

Directions:

1. In a substantial bowl, mix ginger, garlic, ½ cup of cilantro, and ¼ cup of oil.

2. Add pork and coat with mixture generously.

3. Refrigerate to marinate for a few hours.

4. Heat a big skillet on medium-high heat.

5. Add pork mixture and stir fry for approximately 4-5 minutes.

6. Transfer the pork right into a bowl.

7. In the same frying pan, heat the remaining oil on medium heat.

8. Add onion and sauté for approximately 3 minutes.

9. Stir in bell pepper and stir fry for about 3 minutes.

10. Stir in pork, lime juice, and remaining cilantro and cook for about 2 minutes.

11. Serve hot.

Nutrition:

Calories: 429;

Fat: 19g;

Phosphorus: 36mg;

Potassium: 57mg;

Sodium: 31mg;

Carbohydrates: 26g;

Fiber: 9g;

Protein: 35g.

36. PORK WITH PINEAPPLE

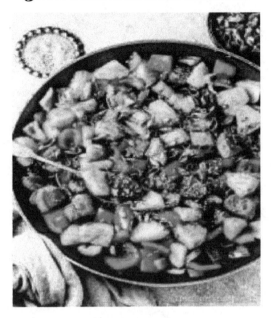

Preparation Time: 15 minutes

Cooking Time: 14 minutes

Serving: 1

Ingredients:

- 2 tablespoons coconut oil
- 1½ pound pork tenderloin, trimmed and cut into bite-sized pieces
- 1 onion, chopped
- 2 minced garlic cloves
- 1 (1-inch) piece fresh ginger, minced

- 20-ounce pineapple, cut into chunks
- 1 large red bell pepper
- ¼ cup fresh pineapple juice
- ¼ cup coconut aminos
- Salt and freshly ground black pepper

Directions:

1. In a substantial skillet, melt coconut oil on high heat.
2. Add pork and stir fry for approximately 4-5 minutes.
3. Transfer the pork into a bowl.
4. In the same frying pan, heat the remaining oil on medium heat.
5. Add onion, garlic, and ginger and sauté for around 2 minutes.
6. Stir in pineapple and bell pepper and stir fry for around 3 minutes.
7. Stir in pork, pineapple juice, and coconut aminos and cook for around 3-4 minutes.
8. Serve hot.

Nutrition:

Calories: 431;

Fat: 10g;

Phosphorus: 36mg;

Potassium: 64mg;

Sodium: 30mg;

Carbohydrates: 22g;

Fiber: 8g;

Protein: 33g.

37. SPICED PORK

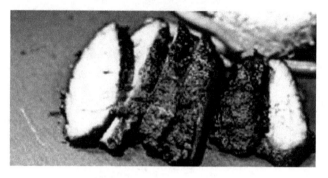

Preparation Time: 15 minutes

Cooking Time: 1 hour 52 minutes

Serving: 1

Ingredients:

- 1 (2-inch) piece fresh ginger, chopped
- 5-10 garlic cloves, chopped
- 1 teaspoon ground cumin
- ½ teaspoon ground turmeric
- 1 tablespoon hot paprika
- 1 tablespoon red pepper flakes
- Salt, to taste
- 2 tablespoons cider vinegar
- 2-pounds pork shoulder, trimmed and cubed into 1½-inch size

- 2 cups domestic hot water, divided
- 1 (1-inch wide) ball tamarind pulp
- ¼ cup olive oil
- 1 teaspoon black mustard seeds, crushed
- 4 green cardamoms
- 5 whole cloves
- 1 (3-inch) cinnamon stick
- 1 cup onion, chopped finely
- 1 large red bell pepper

Directions:

1. In a food processor, add ginger, garlic, cumin, turmeric, paprika, red pepper flakes, salt, and cider vinegar, and pulse till smooth.

2. Transfer the mixture into a large bowl.

3. Add pork and coat it with the mixture generously.

4. Keep aside, covered for around an hour at room temperature.

5. In a bowl, pour 1 cup of warm water and tamarind and keep aside till water cools.

6. With the hands, crush the tamarind to extract the pulp.

7. Add remaining cup of hot water and mix till well combined.

8. Through a fine sieve, strain the tamarind juice in a bowl.

9. In a skillet, heat oil on medium-high heat.

10. Add mustard seeds, green cardamoms, cloves, and cinnamon stick and sauté for about 4 minutes.

11. Add onion and sauté for around 5 minutes.

12. Add pork and stir fry for approximately 6 minutes.

13. Stir in tamarind juice and let it come to a boil.

14. Reduce the heat to medium-low and simmer for 1½ hours.

15. Stir in bell pepper and cook for about 7 minutes.

Nutrition:

Calories: 435;

Fat: 16g;

Phosphorus: 28mg;

Potassium: 64mg;

Sodium: 19mg;

Carbohydrates: 27g;

Fiber: 3g;

Protein: 39g.

38. PORK CHILI

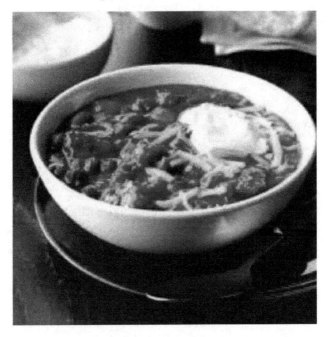

Preparation Time: 15 minutes

Cooking Time: 1 hour

Serving: 1

Ingredients:

- 2 tablespoons extra-virgin organic olive oil

- 2-pound ground pork

- 1 medium red bell pepper

- 1 medium onion, chopped

- 5 garlic cloves, chopped finely

- 1 (2-inch) part of hot pepper, minced

- 1 tablespoon ground cumin

- 1 teaspoon ground turmeric

- 3 tablespoon chili powder

- ½ teaspoon chipotle chili powder

- Salt and freshly ground black pepper

- 1 cup chicken broth

- 1 (28-ounce) can fire-roasted crushed tomatoes

- 2 medium Bok choy heads, sliced

- 1 avocado, peeled, pitted, and chopped

Directions:

1. In a sizable pan, heat oil on medium heat.

2. Add pork and stir fry for about 5 minutes.

3. Add bell pepper, onion, garlic, hot pepper, and spices and stir fry for approximately 5 minutes.

4. Add broth and tomatoes and convey with a boil.

5. Stir in Bok choy and cook, covered for approximately twenty minutes.

6. Uncover and cook for approximately 20 minutes to half an hour.

7. Serve hot while using a topping of avocado.

Nutrition:

Calories: 402;

Fat: 9g;

Phosphorus: 20mg;

Potassium: 156mg;

Sodium: 34mg;

Carbohydrates: 18g;

Fiber: 6g;

Protein: 32g.

39. GROUND PORK WITH WATER CHESTNUTS

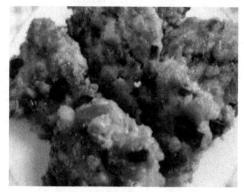

Preparation Time: 15 minutes

Cooking Time: 12 minutes

Serving: 1

Ingredients:

- 1 tablespoon plus 1 teaspoon coconut oil
- 1 tablespoon fresh ginger, minced
- 1 bunch scallion chopped
- 1-pound lean ground pork
- Salt, to taste
- 1 tablespoon 5-spice powder
- 1 (18-ounce) can water chestnuts, drained and chopped
- 1 tablespoon organic honey
- 2 tablespoons fresh lime juice

Directions:

1. In a big heavy-bottomed skillet, heat oil on high heat.

2. Add ginger and scallion whites and sauté for approximately ½-1½ minutes.

3. Add pork and cook for approximately 4-5 minutes.

4. Drain the extra fat from the skillet.

5. Add salt and 5-spice powder and cook for approximately 2-3 minutes.

6. Add scallion greens and remaining ingredients and cook, stirring continuously for about 1-2 minutes.

Nutrition:

Calories: 520;

Fat: 30g;

Phosphorus: 20mg;

Potassium: 120mg;

Sodium: 9mg;

Carbohydrates: 37g;

Fiber: 4g;

Protein: 25g.

40. Hearty Meatloaf

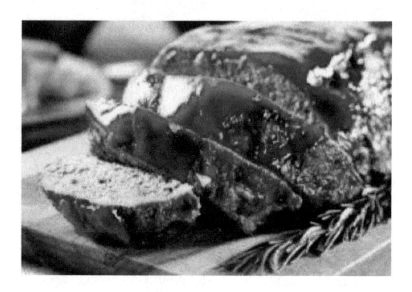

Preparation Time: 10 minutes

Cooking Time: 45-50 minutes

Serving: 1

Ingredients:

- 1 large egg

- 2 tablespoons chopped fresh basil

- 1 teaspoon chopped fresh thyme

- 1 teaspoon chopped fresh parsley

- ¼ teaspoon black pepper (ground)

- 1 pound 95% lean ground beef

- ½ cup breadcrumbs
- ½ cup chopped sweet onion
- 1 teaspoon white vinegar
- ¼ teaspoon garlic powder
- 1 tablespoon brown sugar

Directions:

1. Preheat an oven to 350F. Grease a loaf pan (9X5-inch) with some cooking spray.

2. In a mixing bowl, add beef, breadcrumbs, onion, egg, basil, thyme, parsley, and black pepper. Combine to mix.

3. Add the mixture to the pan.

4. Take another mixing bowl; add brown sugar, vinegar, and garlic powder. Combine to mix well.

5. Add brown sugar mixture over the meat mixture.

6. Bake for about 50 minutes until golden brown.

7. Serve warm.

Nutrition:

Calories: 118;

Fat: 3g;

Phosphorus: 127mg;

Potassium: 203mg;

Sodium: 106mg;

Carbohydrates: 8g;

Protein: 12g.

41. CHICKEN WITH MUSHROOMS

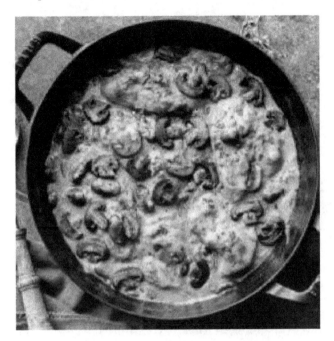

Preparation Time: 15 minutes

Cooking Time: 45 minutes

Serving: 2

Ingredients:

- 2 tablespoons light sour cream

- ¼ cup all-purpose flour

- 1 cup no salt added chicken broth

- 1 tablespoon Dijon mustard

- ¼ teaspoon dried thyme

- 4 chicken breasts

- 1½ cups mushrooms, quartered

- 1 tablespoon non-hydrogenated margarine

- Fresh ground pepper and chopped fresh parsley

- 3 chopped green onions

Directions:

1. Mix 2 tablespoon of chicken broth, mustard, sour cream, and two teaspoon flour. Set aside.

2. Sprinkle chicken with pepper and thyme. Dredge in flour.

3. Melt margarine on medium-low heat in a large non-stick pan. Cook chicken for 15-20 minutes per side. Remove from heat and keep warm.

4. Add mushrooms to another pan. Surge the heat and boil for 3 minutes.

5. Add sour cream mixture and green onions and cook until thickened.

6. Pour over chicken. Garnish with parsley and pepper.

Nutrients:

Protein 25.4g;

Phosphorus: 29mg;

Potassium: 142mg;

Sodium: 17mg;

Carbohydrates 5g;

Fat 4g;

Calories 161

42. Roasted Citrus Chicken

Preparation Time: 20 minutes

Cooking Time: 60 minutes

Servings: 8

Ingredients:

- 1 - Tablespoon olive oil
- 2 - cloves garlic, minced
- 1 - teaspoon Italian seasoning
- ½ - teaspoon black pepper
- 8 - chicken thighs
- 2 - cups chicken broth, reduced-sodium
- 3 - Tablespoons lemon juice
- ½ - large chicken breast for one chicken thigh

Directions:

1. Warm oil in a huge skillet.

2. Include garlic and seasonings.

3. Include chicken bosoms and dark-colored all sides.

4. Spot chicken in the moderate cooker and include the chicken soup.

5. Cook on LOW heat for 6 to 8hours

6. Include lemon juice toward the part of the bargain time.

Nutrition:

Calories: 265

Fat: 19g

Protein: 21g

Carbs: 1g

43. CHICKEN WITH ASIAN VEGETABLES

Preparation Time: 10minutes

Cooking Time: 20 minutes

Servings: 8

Ingredients:

- 2 - Tablespoons canola oil
- 6 - boneless chicken breasts
- 1 - cup low-sodium chicken broth
- 3 - Tablespoons reduced-sodium soy sauce
- ¼ - teaspoon crushed red pepper flakes
- 1 - garlic clove, crushed
- 1 - can (8ounces) water chestnuts, sliced and rinsed (optional)
- ½ - cup sliced green onions
- 1 - cup chopped red or green bell pepper

- 1 - cup chopped celery
- ¼ - cup cornstarch
- 1/3 - cup water
- 3 - cups cooked white rice
- ½ - large chicken breast for one chicken thigh

Directions:

1. Warm oil in a skillet and dark-colored chicken on all sides.

2. Add chicken to a slow cooker with the remainder of the fixings aside from cornstarch and water.

3. Spread and cook on LOW for 6 to 8hours

4. Following 6-8 hours, independently blend cornstarch and cold water until smooth. Gradually include into the moderate cooker.

5. At that point, turn on high for about 15mins until thickened. Don't close the top on the moderate cooker to enable steam to leave.

6. Serve Asian blend over rice.

Nutrition:

Calories: 415

Fat: 20g

Protein: 20g

Carbs: 36g

44. CHICKEN ADOBO

Preparation Time: 10 minutes

Cooking Time: 1hour and 40 minutes

Servings: 6

Ingredients:

- 4 - medium yellow onions, halved and thinly sliced
- 4 - medium garlic cloves, smashed and peeled
- 1 - (5-inch) piece fresh ginger, cut into
- 1 - inch pieces
- 1 - bay leaf
- 3 - pounds bone-in chicken thighs
- 3 - Tablespoons reduced-sodium soy sauce
- ¼ - cup rice vinegar (not seasoned)
- 1 - Tablespoon granulated sugar
- ½ - teaspoon freshly ground black pepper

Directions:

1. Spot the onions, garlic, ginger, and narrows leaf in an even layer in the slight cooker.

2. Take out and do away with the pores and skin from the chicken.

3. Organize the hen in an even layer over the onion mixture.

4. Whisk the soy sauce, vinegar, sugar, and pepper collectively in a medium bowl and pour it over the fowl.

5. Spread and prepare dinner on LOW for 8hours

6. Evacuate and take away the ginger portions and inlet leaf.

7. Present with steamed rice.

Nutrition:

Calories318

Fat: 9g

Protein: 14g

Carbs: 44g

45. CHICKEN AND VEGGIE SOUP

Preparation Time: 15 minutes

Cooking Time: 25 minutes

Servings: 8

Ingredients:

- 4 - cups cooked and chopped chicken
- 7 - cups reduced-sodium chicken broth
- 1 - pound froze white corn
- 1 - medium onion diced
- 4 - cloves garlic minced
- 2 - carrots peeled and diced
- 2 - celery stalks chopped
- 2 - teaspoons oregano
- 2 - teaspoon curry powder
- $1/2$ - teaspoon black pepper

Directions:

1. Include all fixings into the moderate cooker.

2. Cook on LOW for 8hours

3. Serve over cooked white rice.

Nutrition:

Calories220

Fat:7g

Protein: 24g

Carbs: 19g

46. TURKEY SAUSAGES

Preparation Time: 10 Minutes

Cooking time: 10 minutes

Servings: 2

Ingredients:

- 1/4 teaspoon salt
- 1/8 teaspoon garlic powder
- 1/8 teaspoon onion powder
- 1 teaspoon fennel seed
- 1 pound 7% fat ground turkey

Directions:

1. Press the fennel seed and put together turkey with fennel seed, garlic and onion powder, and salt in a small cup.

2. Cover the bowl and refrigerate overnight.

3. Prepare the turkey with seasoning into different portions with a circle form and press them into patties ready to be cooked.

4. Cook at medium heat until browned.

5. Cook it for 1 to 2 minutes per side and serve them hot. Enjoy!

Nutrition:

Calories: 55

Protein: 7 g

Sodium: 70 mg

Potassium: 105 mg

Phosphorus: 75 mg

47. SMOKY TURKEY CHILI

Preparation Time: 5 minutes

Cooking Time: 45 minutes

Servings: 8

Ingredients:

- 12ounce lean ground turkey
- 1/2 red onion, chopped
- 2 cloves garlic, crushed and chopped
- ½ teaspoon of smoked paprika
- ½ teaspoon of chili powder
- ½ teaspoon of dried thyme
- ¼ cup reduced-sodium beef stock
- ½ cup of water

- 1 ½ cups baby spinach leaves, washed
- 3 wheat tortillas

Directions:

1. Brown the ground beef in a dry skillet over medium-high heat.

2. Add in the red onion and garlic.

3. Sauté the onion until it goes clear.

4. Transfer the contents of the skillet to the slow cooker.

5. Add the remaining ingredients and simmer on low for 30–45 minutes.

6. Stir through the spinach for the last few minutes to wilt.

7. Slice tortillas and gently toast under the broiler until slightly crispy.

8. Serve on top of the turkey chili.

Nutrition:

Calories: 93.5

Protein: 8g

Carbohydrates: 3g

Fat: 5.5g

Cholesterol: 30.5mg

Sodium: 84.5mg

Potassium: 142.5mg

Phosphorus: 92.5mg

Calcium: 29mg

Fiber: 0.5g

48. ROSEMARY CHICKEN

Preparation Time: 10 Minutes

Cooking time: 10 minutes

Servings: 2

Ingredients:

- 2 zucchinis
- 1 carrot
- 1 teaspoon dried rosemary
- 4 chicken breasts
- 1/2 bell pepper
- 1/2 red onion
- 8 garlic cloves
- Olive oil
- 1/4 tablespoon ground pepper

Directions:

1. Prepare the oven and preheat it at 375 °F (or 200°C).

2. Slice both zucchini and carrots and add bell pepper, onion, garlic, and put everything adding oil in a 13" x 9" pan.

3. Spread the pepper over everything and roast for about 10 minutes.

4. Meanwhile, lift the chicken skin and spread black pepper and rosemary on the flesh.

5. Take away the vegetable pan from the oven and add the chicken, returning it to the oven for about 30 more minutes. Serve and enjoy!

Nutrition:

Calories: 215

Protein: 28 g

Sodium: 105 mg

Potassium: 580 mg

Phosphorus: 250 mg

49. AVOCADO-ORANGE GRILLED CHICKEN

Preparation Time: 20 minutes

Cooking Time: 60 minutes

Servings: 4

Ingredients:

- ¼ cup fresh lime juice
- ¼ cup minced red onion
- 1 avocado
- 1 cup low-fat yogurt
- 1 small red onion, sliced thinly

- 1 tablespoon honey
- 2 oranges, peeled and sectioned
- 2 tablespoons. chopped cilantro
- 4 pieces of 4-6ounce boneless, skinless chicken breasts
- Pepper and salt to taste

Directions:

1. In a large bowl, mix honey, cilantro, minced red onion, and yogurt.

2. Submerge chicken into mixture and marinate for at least 30 minutes.

3. Grease grate and preheat grill to medium-high fire.

4. Remove chicken from marinade and season with pepper and salt.

5. Grill for 6 minutes per side or until chicken is cooked and juices run clear.

6. Meanwhile, peel the avocado and discard the seed. Chop avocados and place them in a bowl. Quickly add lime juice and toss avocado to coat well with juice.

7. Add cilantro, thinly sliced onions, and oranges into a bowl of avocado, mix well.

8. Serve grilled chicken and avocado dressing on the side.

Nutrition:

Calories: 209

Carbs: 26g;

Protein: 8g;

Fats: 10g;

Phosphorus: 157mg;

Potassium: 548mg;

Sodium: 125mg

50. HERBS AND LEMONY ROASTED CHICKEN

Preparation Time: 15 minutes

Cooking Time: 1 ½ hour

Servings: 8

Ingredients:

- ½ teaspoon ground black pepper
- ½ teaspoon mustard powder
- ½ teaspoon salt
- 1 3-lb whole chicken
- 1 teaspoon garlic powder

- 2 lemons
- 2 tablespoons. olive oil
- 2 teaspoons. Italian seasoning

Directions:

1. In a small bowl, mix well black pepper, garlic powder, mustard powder, and salt.

2. Rinse chicken well and slice off giblets.

3. In a greased 9 x 13 baking saucer, put the chicken and add 1 ½ teaspoon. of seasoning made earlier inside the chicken and rub the remaining seasoning around the chicken.

4. In a small bowl, mix olive oil and juice from 2 lemons. Drizzle over chicken.

5. Bake chicken in a preheated 3500F oven until juices run clear, around 1 ½ hour. Every once in a while, baste the chicken with its juices.

Nutrition:

Calories: 190;

Carbs: 2g;

Protein: 35g;

Fats: 9g;

Phosphorus: 341mg;

Potassium: 439mg;

Sodium: 328mg

51. GROUND CHICKEN & PEAS CURRY

Preparation Time: 15 minutes

Cooking Time: 6-10 minutes

Servings: 3-4

Ingredients:

- 3 tablespoons essential olive oil
- 2 bay leaves
- 2 onions, ground to some paste
- ½ tablespoon garlic paste
- ½ tablespoon ginger paste
- 2 tomatoes, chopped finely
- 1 tablespoon ground cumin
- 1 tablespoon ground coriander
- 1 teaspoon ground turmeric
- 1 teaspoon red chili powder
- Salt, to taste
- 1-pound lean ground chicken
- 2 cups frozen peas

- 1½ cups water
- 1-2 teaspoons garam masala powder

Directions:

1. In a deep-frying pan, heat oil with medium heat.

2. Add bay leaves and sauté for approximately half a minute.

3. Add onion paste and sauté for approximately 3-4 minutes.

4. Add garlic and ginger paste and sauté for around 1-1½ minutes.

5. Add tomatoes and spices and cook, occasionally stirring, for about 3-4 minutes.

6. Stir in chicken and cook for about 4-5 minutes.

7. Stir in peas and water and bring to a boil on high heat.

8. Reduce the heat to low and simmer for approximately 5-8 minutes or till the desired doneness.

9. Stir in garam masala and remove from heat.

10. Serve hot.

Nutrition:

Calories: 450,

Fat: 10g,

Carbohydrates: 19g,

Fiber: 6g,

Protein: 38g

52. CHICKEN MEATBALLS CURRY

Preparation Time: 20 minutes

Cooking Time: 25 minutes

Servings: 3-4

Ingredients:

For Meatballs:

- 1-pound lean ground chicken
- 1 tablespoon onion paste
- 1 teaspoon fresh ginger paste
- 1 teaspoon garlic paste
- 1 green chili, chopped finely
- 1 tablespoon fresh cilantro leaves, chopped
- 1 teaspoon ground coriander

- ½ teaspoon cumin seeds
- ½ teaspoon red chili powder
- ½ teaspoon ground turmeric
- Salt, to taste

For Curry:

- 3 tablespoons extra-virgin olive oil
- ½ teaspoon cumin seeds
- 1 (1-inch) cinnamon stick
- 3 whole cloves
- 3 whole green cardamoms
- 1 whole black cardamom
- 2 onions, chopped
- 1 teaspoon fresh ginger, minced
- 1 teaspoon garlic, minced
- 4 whole tomatoes, chopped finely
- 2 teaspoons ground coriander
- 1 teaspoon garam masala powder
- ½ teaspoon ground nutmeg
- ½ teaspoon red chili powder
- ½ teaspoon ground turmeric
- Salt, to taste
- 1 cup of water
- Chopped fresh cilantro for garnishing

Directions:

1. For meatballs in a substantial bowl, add all ingredients and mix till well combined.

2. Make small equal-sized meatballs from the mixture.

3. In a big deep skillet, heat oil on medium heat.

4. Add meatballs and fry approximately 3-5 minutes or till browned from all sides.

5. Transfer the meatballs to a bowl.

6. In the same skillet, add cumin seeds, cinnamon stick, cloves, green cardamom, and black cardamom and sauté for approximately 1 minute.

7. Add onions and sauté for around 4-5 minutes.

8. Add ginger and garlic paste then sauté for approximately 1 minute.

9. Add tomato and spices and cook, crushing with the back of the spoon for approximately 2-3 minutes.

10. Add water and meatballs and provide to a boil.

11. Reduce heat to low.

12. Simmer for approximately 10 minutes.

13. Serve hot with all the garnishing of cilantro.

Nutrition:

Calories: 421,

Fat: 8g,

Carbohydrates: 18g,

Fiber: 5g,

Protein: 34g

30 Days Meal Plan

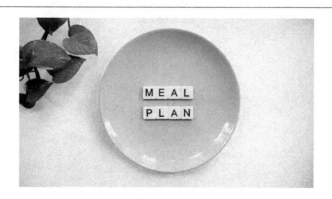

Days	Breakfast	Lunch	Dinner	Desserts/ Smoothies
1	Asparagus Frittata	Dolmas Wrap	Creamy Crab Over Salmon	Spiced Peaches
2	Poached Eggs with Cilantro Butter	Salad al Tonno	Slow-Cooked Beef Brisket	Pumpkin Cheesecake Bar
3	Chorizo and Egg Tortilla	Arlecchino Rice Salad	Pork Souvlaki	Blueberry Mini Muffins
4	Cottage Cheese Pancakes	Greek Salad	Open-Faced Beef Stir-Up	Vanilla Custard

5	Egg in a Hole	Sautéed Chickpea and Lentil Mix	Grilled Steak with Cucumber Salsa	Chocolate Chip Cookies
6	German Pancakes	Baked Vegetables Soup	Beef Brisket	Baked Peaches with Cream Cheese
7	Mushroom and Red Pepper Omelet	Pesto Chicken Salad	Apricot and Lamb Tagine	Bread Pudding
8	Apple and Zucchini Bread	Falafel	Lamb Shoulder with Zucchini and Eggplant	Strawberry Ice Cream
9	Spicy Corn Bread	Israeli Pasta Salad	Beef Chili	Cinnamon Custard
10	Breakfast Casserole	Artichoke Matzo Mina	Skirt Steak Glazed with Bourbon	Raspberry Brule

11	Grilled Veggie and Cheese Bagel	Shrimp Paella	Beef Pot Roast	Tart Apple Granita
12	Cauliflower Tortilla	Salmon and Pesto Salad	Grilled Lamb Chops	Lemon-Lime Sherbet
13	Eggs Benedict	Baked Fennel and Garlic Sea Bass	Lamb and Pineapple Kebabs	Pavlova with Peaches
14	Cranberry and Apple Oatmeal	Lemon, Garlic & Cilantro Tuna and Rice	Baked Meatballs and Scallions	Tropical Vanilla Snow Cone
15	Blueberry Breakfast Smoothie	Cod & Green Bean Risotto	Pork with Bell Pepper	Rhubarb Crumble
16	Apple Sauce Cream Toast	Mixed Pepper Stuffed River Trout	Pork with Pineapple	Gingerbread Loaf

17	Waffles	Haddock & Buttered Leeks	Pork Chili	Elegant Lavender Cookies
18	Egg Whites and Veggie Bake	Thai Spiced Halibut	Ground Pork with Water Chestnuts	Carob Angel Food Cake
19	Green Breakfast Soup	Homemade Tuna Niçoise	Hearty Meatloaf	Old-Fashioned Apple Kuchen
20	Peach Berry Parfait	Monk-Fish Curry	Chicken with Mushrooms	Almonds & Blueberries Smoothie
21	Open-Faced Bagel Breakfast Sandwich	Oregon Tuna Patties	Roasted Citrus Chicken	Almonds and Zucchini Smoothie
22	Bulgur Bowl with Strawberries and Walnuts	Fish Chowder	Chicken with Asian Vegetables	Avocado with Walnut Butter Smoothie

23	Overnight Oats Three Ways	Broiled Sesame Cod	Chicken Adobo	Baby Spinach and Dill Smoothie
24	Buckwheat Pancakes	Tuna Salad with Cranberries	Chicken and Veggie Soup	Blueberries and Coconut Smoothie
25	Avocado Egg Bake	Zucchini Cups with Dill Cream and Smoked Tuna	Turkey Sausages	Collard Greens and Cucumber Smoothie
26	Broccoli Basil Quiche	Creamy Smoked Tuna Macaroni	Smoky Turkey Chili	Creamy Dandelion Greens and Celery Smoothie
27	Hawaiian Chicken Salad	Asparagus and Smoked Tuna Salad	Rosemary Chicken	Dark Turnip Greens Smoothie

28	Grated Carrot Salad with Lemon-Dijon Vinaigrette	Spicy Tuna Salad Sandwiches	Avocado-Orange Grilled Chicken	Butter Pecan and Coconut Smoothie
29	Tuna Macaroni Salad	Spanish Tuna	Herbs and Lemony Roasted Chicken	Fresh Cucumber, Kale, and Raspberry Smoothie
30	Couscous Salad	Fish with Vegetables	Ground Chicken & Peas Curry	Happy Heart Energy Bites

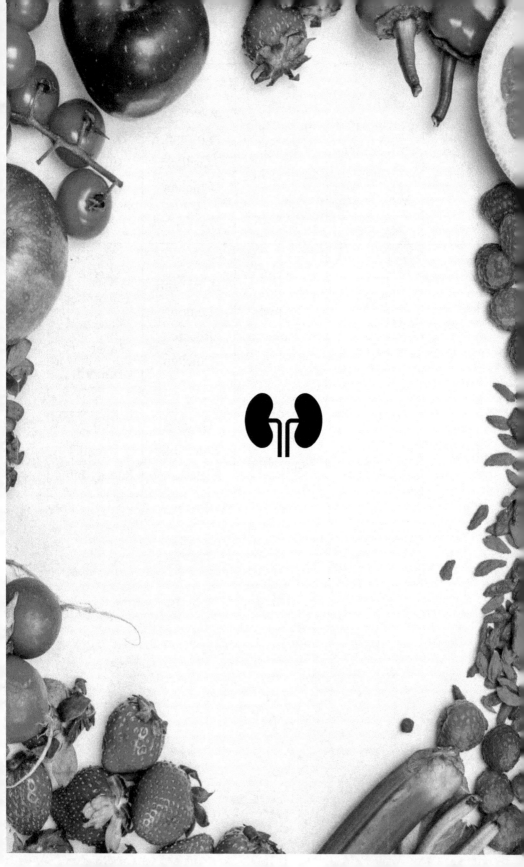

TIPS

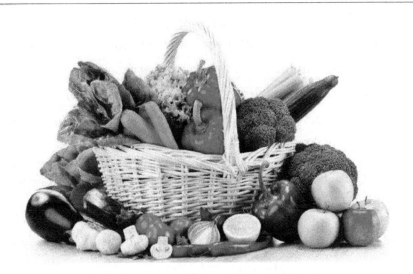

TIPS ON CONTROLLING YOUR PHOSPHORUS

Phosphorus is a well-known mineral that the body can get rid of through the urine, thanks to healthy kidneys. However, if kidneys malfunction, phosphorus starts building up in the blood vessels, resulting in many serious health problems. The kidneys' inability to remove extra phosphorus from the body can cause several pains like heart calcification, joint pain, and easily broken bones.

Phosphorus has always been related to the bone's health, and together with calcium, bones are indispensable for maintaining healthy bones. And to keep the level of phosphorus balanced in your body, you should carefully watch the foods you eat like meats, poultry, fish, beans, nuts, and dairy products. Phosphorus is more likely to be found in animal foods and plant foods, yet our body absorbs the phosphorus we get from animal foods more than from plant foods.

The phosphorus added to certain foods is not as healthy as we can imagine because it comes in the form of preservatives and additives, and it can be found in fast and junk foods. We might not know that our body absorbs the phosphorus that we get from food additives. Hence, avoiding additives is the best way we can use to lower the intake of phosphorus additives. You should always check the facts on each food label you buy and search for the "Phos" to know which contains more phosphorous.

To maintain a balanced level of phosphorous and to keep it under control; here is what you should do:

Limit the consumption of foods like poultry, meats, fish, and dairy

- Limit the intake of certain dairy products like yogurt and cheese; you should not exceed 4 oz. per serving
- Avoid black beans, lima beans, red beans, garbanzo beans, white beans, and black-eyed peas.
- Avoid unrefined, whole, and dark grains.
- Stay away from refrigerator dough
- Avoid dried fruits and vegetables
- Avoid chocolate
- Avoid dark-colored sodas
- The renal diet limits the intake of phosphorus to 1000mg per day

TIPS ON CONTROLLING YOUR PROTEIN

Protein makes an essential element of our growth, and it plays a vital role in maintaining our body mass. Besides, proteins can help us fight any infection that can threaten our bodies. And while proteins are essential for our health, excessive consumption may lead to undesirable and even threatening results. Eating more than your body needs can hasten the deterioration of your kidneys.

Therefore, maintaining a moderate and balanced intake of proteins can keep your body healthy, and it can prevent kidney failure. Furthermore, when your kidneys cannot function very well, they start leaking protein into your urine, which can lead to many unpleasant side effects like a change in taste, loss of appetite, nausea, and even fatigue.

In a few words, protein is essential for the growth and maintenance of our health, and it is substantial in healing wounds, fighting all infections, and providing our body with the energy it needs. Nevertheless, it's significant to keep the level of proteins in our bodies balanced.

To make sure that our kidneys are not stressed by the proteins we eat, we should consume high-quality proteins. And we should make sure that we eat about 7 to 8 oz. of protein per day. 1 Egg equals 1 oz. of protein.

Pork, beef, turkey, veal, chicken, and eggs have high amounts of protein.

TIPS ON CONTROLLING YOUR FLUID INTAKE

When your kidneys function correctly, they can get rid of the fluids that enter your body. However, when our kidneys are not working correctly and, our body might not be able to get rid of the juices as it used to. The build-up of fluids in our body can lead to swelling, high blood pressure, and even shortness of breath.

Therefore, we should limit our intake of fluids and keep it under control to avoid dialysis at a specific step. There are many foods high in water, like ice cream, sauces, rice pudding, gravy, and custard. You should cut down on some food packed with water and avoid some other foods as well. Moreover, people who suffer from kidney diseases and consume high levels of fluids may experience pressure on the heart and the lungs.

And Here Are Some Tips with Which You Can Restrict the Intake of Fluids:

1. Use 1 cup or glass to divide your fluid intake per day. You can also write a record of your fluid intake.
2. Always avoid any salty food and never add extra salt to your meals.
3. Avoid processed meats, fast foods, and canned foods
4. You can add lemon juice to the water you want to drink instead
5. You can have a mouthwash from time to time
6. Avoid overheating
7. Maintain your blood sugar at a balanced level

ARE YOU EATING OUT?

You can still enjoy your favorite restaurant or cuisines! Look out for small or half portions and ask your server for your foods to be cooked without extra salts, butter or sauces. Avoid fried foods. Instead, embrace poached or grilled food.

If you know you are going out to eat, plan. Look at the restaurant's menu beforehand and decide what you will order to avoid anxiety or stress on the night! Be sure to take your phosphorus binders if they have been prescribed to you. Take them with your meal instead of waiting until you get home.

FAQs

Q: How Can I Figure Out If a Food Label or Recipe Is Low in Potassium and What Is the Maximum Daily Limit?

A: When following a renal diet, you ideally want to make sure that potassium levels are below 250mg/per serving or up to 7% of the food's total nutritional value. If the food/recipe indicates less than 100 mg of potassium per serving, this means that it's shallow in potassium. However, a moderate rate of up to 250 mg per serving is acceptable, as long as you don't consume any other foods throughout the day with middle or high potassium levels, e.g., between 250-400 mg/serving.

Q: Can One Lose Weight During a Renal Diet?

A: If you wish to lose extra weight for health or fitness reasons, you can follow a renal diet plan that is preferably high in fats, and fiber foods, e.g., forest fruits, cabbage, etc. make sure that your daily calorie intake does not exceed 2000 calories, and any foods you choose are low in sodium and potassium to keep bloating and fluid build-up under control. It would help if you took several calories, though, depends on your age, gender, health status, and weight goal that you wish to achieve. If you want to lose weight and your renal diet plan, it's better to discuss the matter with an expert dietician or nutritionist.

Q: Does My CKD Stage Count When Following a Renal Diet?

A: Absolutely! In earlier stages (up to the third stage), it is acceptable to consume low to moderate amounts of sodium, potassium, and phosphorus, while your fluid intake should be up to 2.5 liters per day. However, when you are in a more advanced renal damage stage, you have further to limit all the above minerals and fluids, e.g., drink up to 2 liters of fluids per day or only up to 150 mg of potassium meal (instead of 250mg). Your doctor or dietician will give you additional guidelines on the exact amounts of each that you need to take daily, based on your current stage of renal disease.

Q: Is It OK to Take Caffeine in a Renal Diet?

A: In most cases and especially during the first three CKD stages, a caffeine-based drink is perfectly fine. You may drink up to 2 cups of coffee or caffeine tea per day without any worries. However, be careful as any extras that you add to your coffee will not only increase calories; they may raise potassium levels as well. Such toppings are whipping cream, caramel syrups, chocolate, etc. Pure coffee or black tea with water and a bit of almond or soy milk isn't an issue, but anything "fortified" should be avoided.

Q: Can I Take Over the Counter Medication When on a Renal Diet?

A: Unfortunately, the vast majority of over the counter medication/painkillers like aspirin and ibuprofen are not indicated for CKD patients. Any drug that belongs in the NSAID (nonsteroidal anti-inflammatory drugs) category should be avoided. According to some studies, NSAIDs can worsen CKD. Some other types of medication are also not indicated for renal patients. If you are currently taking any other medicines, it would be wise to consult your doctor to find out whether they are OK for kidney function or not.

CONCLUSION:

Kidney disease now ranks as the 18th deadliest condition in the world. In the United States alone, it is reported that over 600,000 Americans succumb to kidney failure.

These stats are alarming, which is why it is necessary to take proper care of your kidneys, starting with a kidney-friendly diet.

In this book, you will learn to create dishes that are healthy, delicious, and easy for your kidneys.

These recipes are ideal for whether you have been diagnosed with a kidney problem or want to prevent any kidney issue.

Regarding your well-being and health, it's a smart thought to see your doctor as frequently as conceivable to ensure you don't run into preventable issues that you needn't get. The kidneys are your body's toxin channel (just like the liver), cleaning the blood of remote substances and toxins that are discharged from things like preservatives in food & other toxins.

At the point when you eat flippantly and fill your body with toxins, either from nourishment, drinks (liquor or alcohol, for instance), or even from the air you inhale (free radicals are in the sun and move through your skin, through messy air, and numerous food sources contain them). In general, your body will convert numerous things that appear to be benign until your body's organs convert them into things like formaldehyde because of a synthetic response and transforming phase.

One case of this is a large portion of those diet sugars utilized in diet soft drinks, for instance. Aspartame transforms into Formaldehyde in the body. These toxins must be expelled, or they can prompt ailment, renal (kidney) failure, malignant growth, & various other painful problems.

This isn't a condition that occurs without any forethought; it is a dynamic issue, and in that it very well may be both found early and treated, diet changed, and settling what is causing the issue is conceivable. It's conceivable to have partial renal failure, yet, as a rule, it requires some time (or downright awful diet for a short time) to arrive at absolute renal failure. You would prefer not to reach total renal failure since this will require standard dialysis treatments to save your life.

Dialysis treatments explicitly clean the blood of waste and toxins in the blood utilizing a machine because your body can no longer carry out the responsibility. Without treatments, you could die an excruciating death. Renal failure can be the consequence of long-haul diabetes, hypertension, unreliable diet, and can stem from other health concerns.

A renal diet is tied in with directing the intake of protein and phosphorus in your eating routine. Restricting your sodium intake is likewise significant. By controlling these two variables, you can control the vast majority of the toxins/waste made by your body, and thus, this enables your kidney to 100% function. If you get this early enough and truly moderate your diets with extraordinary consideration, you could avert all-out renal failure. If you get this early, you can take out the issue completely.

CPSIA information can be obtained
at www.ICGtesting.com
Printed in the USA
LVHW081656030321
679517LV00005BA/207